CONSULTATION SKILLS FOR THE MRCGP

SECOND EDITION

This item comes with accompanying CD/DVD's

Please ask at the library enquiry desk for details.

CONSULTATION SKILLS FOR THE MRCGP

SECOND EDITION

P. NAIDOO

MBChB, MRCGP, DRCOG, DFFP, Dip Occ, MSc
GP in Oxfordshire

AND

C. MONKLEY

MBBS, DRCOG, MSc (Sports Medicine), MRCGP, FFSEM (UK),
GP in the Defence Medical Services

Scion

Second edition published 2012

© **Scion Publishing Ltd, 2012**

First edition published 2009 and reprinted 2010, 2011

A CIP catalogue record for this book is available from the British Library.

ISBN 978 1 904842 96 5

Scion Publishing Limited
The Old Hayloft, Vantage Business Park, Bloxham Road,
Banbury, Oxfordshire, OX16 9UX, UK
www.scionpublishing.com

Important Note from the Publisher
The information contained within this book was obtained by Scion Publishing Limited from sources believed by us to be reliable. However, while every effort has been made to ensure its accuracy, no responsibility for loss or injury whatsoever occasioned to any person acting or refraining from action as a result of information contained herein can be accepted by the authors or publishers.

The reader should remember that medicine is a constantly evolving science and while the authors and publishers have ensured that all dosages, applications and practices are based on current indications, there may be specific practices which differ between communities. You should always follow the guidelines laid down by the manufacturers of specific products and the relevant authorities in the country in which you are practising.

Typeset by Phoenix Photosetting, Chatham, Kent, UK
Printed by the Complete Product Company, Malmesbury, Wiltshire, UK

Contents

Contents

Preface

This book is written as a companion guide to *Cases and Concepts for the new MRCGP*, 2nd edition (2009). The aim is to help readers pull together the knowledge and communication skills required for success in the consultation components of the MRCGP exam, namely Clinical Skills Assessment (CSA) and Clinical Observation Tool (COT). The book does this in three ways:

- by demonstrating some of the required consultation skills on the accompanying DVD
- by identifying and teaching these skills in the case write-ups
- by giving candidates 'practice cases' on which to practise, either alone or in small groups

The book and DVD are meant to be interactive. The DVD features 13 GP consultations and readers are asked if the doctor on the DVD:

- asked the right questions, at the right time, in the right way
- performed the right examination correctly
- communicated in a precise, understandable and sensitive manner

In the DVD cases that are marked according to a CSA marking schedule, readers are referred to various sources of information so that they have adequate knowledge to make judgements. In all the cases, additional medical information is provided to clarify the management decisions and justify the weighting of the accompanying marking schedule. If readers feel that the doctor's performance in a particular area is inadequate, they are invited to suggest how they would improve performance. Group work can be quite useful in this regard.

Once candidates learn from the DVD, they are presented with 20 complete cases designed to aid them in CSA preparation and COT discussions. Each of the 20 cases features detailed analysis to demonstrate to candidates an ordered, step-wise approach to data gathering, clinical management and interpersonal skills. It is important to learn and practise these skills, but the trainee who tries to practise every potential examination case to get the 'answer right' is embarking on a long and exhausting journey. It may be a more efficient use of time to recognise a type of case and to have a methodical approach.

For example, some cases are written to be ethical dilemmas; others are cases where the patient presents with a request, i.e. the solution which they think is the answer to their clinical problem. If you recognise the type of case (for example, patient presents with a specific request), work out what you need to demonstrate (for example, thorough assessment of the underlying problem, a choice of options the patient may not have considered, arguments for and against the specific request). If you recognise the type of case and roll out your methodical approach, you do not have to practise every mock CSA case written around this permutation. Think of skilled learner drivers who have practised hill starts, urban and rural traffic – they do not try to drive down every possible road before the driving test. Success depends on recognising a hill start and deploying your pre-planned strategy, which you have practised on several previous occasions.

With this in mind, the book is useful to Specialist Trainees (ST) in general practice right from the start of their training.

- ST1s will find DVD cases 1–7 most useful.
- ST2s, reading the analysis and discussion in the long cases, will be prepared for COT discussions.
- ST3s preparing for the CSA are directed to DVD cases 8–13 and the final section of the book, Practice Cases, which provides examples of typical CSA questions and focuses on cases not previously covered in *Cases and Concepts for the new MRCGP*. There is greater coverage of paediatric and telephone consultations, dealing with lists, breaking bad news, and home visits.

Good luck with your studying!

Dr P Naidoo
March 2012

Acknowledgments

Thank you to my trainees – you have been an inspiration, challenge and pleasure to teach.

The Defence Deanery: thank you for electing me as the GPEC trainer rep in 2010. It was a fascinating experience.

Robin: thanks for inviting me to teach on Highlands and Islands. It was hugely enjoyable, except for the early morning run.

Finally, to my husband Anton – of course you can have Sky Sports. Life is much richer for watching decent southern hemisphere rugby.

Dedication

This book is dedicated to my mother who has enjoyed teaching for more than 40 years, a hard act to follow.

Analysing consultation skills: the DVD

The aim of the DVD (attached to the inside back cover) is to model for candidates the communication skills required for effective consultation in the COT and CSA. There are thirteen cases in total. Video cases one to seven are analysed using the COT template. Video cases eight to thirteen are accompanied by a CSA marking grid to give the viewer a chance to assess the doctor's performance.

Each of the 13 video cases comprises the following sections.
- *'Brief to the doctor'*, with a summary of the patient's relevant details, including any recent test results. The 'locum' doctor, like the CSA candidate, is provided with the patient's basic background at the start of clinic.
- *'Tasks for the doctor'*: in video cases one to seven, the doctor is tasked to observe the useful consultation skills this case illustrates and to comment on whether any important aspects of the consultation are omitted. In video cases eight to thirteen, the candidate is informed about the examiner's thought processes, which explains the weighting of the accompanying marking grid.
- *'Approach to be taken'*: a review of the doctor's approach is provided in video cases one to seven, with an explanation of consultation behaviours demonstrated and missed. In video cases eight to thirteen, a CSA marking grid is provided to enable candidates to mark the DVD cases themselves.
- *'Debrief'*: each debrief highlights the communication techniques that can be learnt from the case.
- Each case ends with suggestions for further reading.

Video cases 1–7
- Read through the case's entire write-up before watching the DVD.
- Look at the 'tasks for the doctor when watching the case' so that you are clear about which specific techniques you are cued to observe.
- Watch the case. You may wish to use a COT *pro forma* to help you to 'mark' the doctor's performance. Please remember, marks are given for the doctor's questioning, examination technique and explanation, and not for the patient's contribution.
- Debrief, either alone, or in a group, consolidating the skills learnt from the case.

Video cases 8–13
- Read through the 'patient summary' and 'tasks for the doctor'.
- Refer to the background information provided – this informs the marking grid.
- While watching the DVD, consult the marking grid and tick when positive or negative indicators are demonstrated.
- Make a global judgement by asking if this doctor, based on this consultation, is fit for independent practice.
- Debrief, preferably in a small group.

COT *pro forma*[1]

A. Data gathering, examination and clinical assessment skills

1. Define the clinical problem:
- What questions do you ask to clarify why the patient has presented today?
- How would you explore the patient's ideas, concerns, expectations and health beliefs?

2. Perform an appropriate physical or mental examination
- What is the appropriate targeted physical or mental state examination?
- Can you perform the examination slickly and sensitively using appropriate medical equipment?

B. Clinical management skills

3. Make an appropriate working diagnosis
- On the basis of probability, what is your working diagnosis?

4. Explain the problem to the patient using appropriate language
- How would you explain the diagnosis to the patient?
- Is your explanation jargon-free, well organised and logical?
- Does it address the patient's concerns and expectations?

5. Provide holistic care and use resources effectively
- Was your management plan informed by national or local guidelines?
- Have you referred appropriately?

6. Prescribe appropriately
- Have you considered drug interactions or discussed side effects?
- Did you check the patient's understanding of the medication?

7. Specify the conditions and interval for follow-up
- Have you safety netted appropriately?

---

1   Adapted from a COT *pro forma* developed by Dr David Chadwick, Springfield Surgery, Oxfordshire.

C. Interpersonal skills: know and treat this patient

8. Achieve rapport
- Have you demonstrated active listening, sensitivity, and empathy?
- Have you used the patient's ideas and beliefs in explanations?
- Have you addressed the patient's specific concerns and expectations?

9. Give the patient the opportunity to be involved in significant management decisions
- Have you involved the patient in decisions?
- Have you negotiated, offered various treatment options or encouraged autonomy and opinions?

Video 1 – Knee pain

Brief to the doctor

Miss AS is a 22 year old woman who presents with knee pain.

Patient summary

Name	AS
Date of birth (Age)	22
Past medical history	Contraception
Repeat medication	Microgynon as directed

Tasks for the doctor when watching the case

The tasks are to:
- take note of the verbal and non-verbal communication the doctor employed to put the patient at ease
- notice how the doctor used a mixture of open and closed questions to take a systematic and detailed history
- comment on the fluency of the doctor's examination
- assess whether the examination findings proved or disproved the doctor's suspicions
- assess whether the patient understood the explanation? How could the doctor have simplified the explanation or checked the patient's understanding?

Review of the doctor's approach

A. Data gathering, examination and clinical assessment skills

1. *Define the clinical problem: clarify why the patient has presented today*
   The doctor:
   - leaned forward, smiled, made good eye contact and nodded appropriately, thereby establishing good rapport
   - asked open questions to explore the problem, such as *"how can I help?"* and *"describe the pain?"*
   - asked closed questions to clarify details about the knee pain: *"do you get pain at other times? Is there giving way? Locking? Is there pain on walking up or down the stairs? Have you injured the knee? Are there problems with other joints?"*

- explored the patient's health understanding by asking *"have you thought about what this might be?"*
- explored the patient's concerns: *"is there anything you are worried about?"*

The doctor could have:

- gained more information on how the knee pain was affecting her job or her activities at home. He could have enquired whether her inability to train affected her interactions with work colleagues.

2. *Performs an appropriate physical or mental examination*
- The knee was examined; hence the examination was appropriate and directed.

The doctor could have:

- asked the patient if she preferred to have a chaperone present
- made the examination more fluent and systematic, following the 'look, feel and move' approach to joint examination

B. Clinical management skills

3. *Make an appropriate working diagnosis*
- The doctor made a working diagnosis of 'problem with the tendon at the knee cap'.
- The case was written to be patello-femoral pain, secondary to excessive foot pronation.

4. *Explain the problem to the patient using appropriate language*
The doctor:
- attempted to explain the diagnosis to the patient using phrases such as *"the ligaments are intact"* and *"there is no fluid in the knee"*
- prescribed ibuprofen and paracetamol appropriately and the doctor specifically asked if the patient knew what the maximum dosages were, thus demonstrating an attempt to enhance concordance

However, the doctor:

- used words such as 'cartilage', 'tendon', 'inflammation' without clarification and the assessor is not sure if the language used was 'appropriate', particularly as the doctor did not specifically confirm the patient's understanding of the diagnosis
- did not give the patient the opportunity to be involved in the management plan, although it is entirely appropriate to prescribe pain medication and refer to physiotherapy

5. *Provide holistic care and use resources effectively*
The doctor:
- was informed by guidelines (www.emedicine.com/ and search for 'patellofemoral syndrome')

However, the assessor is unsure if:

- holistic care was provided: the issue of training for a marathon was not addressed
- resources were used effectively as the patient's views on taking medication and attending physiotherapy were not sought

6. *Prescribe appropriately*
   The doctor:

   - checked the patient's understanding of the amounts of medication required

7. *Specify the conditions and interval for follow-up*
   The doctor could have:

   - highlighted the importance of proper assessments for suitable footwear
   - specified when he would like to review the patient again, such as *"I expect this condition to improve with physiotherapy but if you make little progress, please see me again"*

C. Interpersonal skills: know and treat this patient

8. *Achieve rapport*
   The doctor:

   - listened attentively to the patient's description of her problem
   - spoke when she stopped – the consultation had a natural cadence
   - empathised with her difficulties in training for the marathon
   - asked if there was anything further the patient required at the end of the consultation

9. *Give the patient the opportunity to be involved in significant management decisions*
   The doctor could have:

   - encouraged autonomy by asking what the patient thought of physiotherapy or non-steroidals

Debrief

- What could you learn from this consultation? How to
  - establish rapport
  - take a systematic and focused history
  - explore the patient's health understanding
  - take steps to enhance concordance
  - be efficient with time
- What questions could you ask to discover the patient's ideas and expectations?
- How would you examine the knee?
- How could you explain the diagnosis of patello-femoral syndrome to the patient?
- How could you involve the patient in the management plan?

Relevant literature

For an excellent website from the University of California, San Diego, detailing the examination of the knee, with video-clips, see http://meded.ucsd.edu/clinicalmed/knee_exam.htm or http://meded.ucsd.edu/clinicalmed/joints.htm and click on 'video showing complete knee exam'

For information on patello-femoral syndrome, see www.emedicine.com/pmr/topic101.htm

Video 2 – Unhappy with last consultation

Brief to the doctor

Mrs SW is a 31 year old woman who saw Dr Brown 2 weeks ago. She is unhappy with her last consultation.

Patient summary

Name	SW
Date of birth (Age)	31
Social and Family History	Married, no children
Past medical history	Sprained ankle 3 years ago
Repeat medication	Marvelon as directed

Consultation note by Dr Brown (2 weeks ago):
'Long list of minor symptoms. Thinks she has diabetes. Urine dipstix negative for glucose. Reassured no diabetes.'

Tasks for the doctor when watching the case

The tasks are to:
- notice how the doctor used open questions to gather a lot of data, followed by summarising to highlight the main problems and indicate to the patient that the doctor had a good grasp of the pertinent issues – this communication style allowed the doctor to structure the consultation
- notice that the open questions were neutral, for example, *"What do you think he did to make you feel like that?"* The non-judgemental questioning style enabled the doctor to obtain information without defending or undermining Dr Brown.
- take note of the doctor's response to an important cue – the patient, early in the consultation, mentioned that symptoms interfered with work; the doctor jotted down the cue, continued with her line of questioning, but a few minutes later asked how the symptoms interfered with work
- comment on how the patient's ideas (on the cause of diabetes), concerns (about a missed early diagnosis) and expectations (of better testing) were elicited

Review of the doctor's approach

A. Data gathering, examination and clinical assessment skills

1. *Define the clinical problem: clarify why the patient has presented today*
   The doctor:
   - established good rapport by greeting the patient at the door, smiling, and inviting her to sit
   - summarised the history at intervals thereby indicating active listening
   - asked open questions to explore the problem, such as *"when you say excessive, what do you mean? Are there any other symptoms? What happens to you when you get irritable?"*
   - asked closed questions to assess the likelihood of diabetes: *"are you passing more urine? Are you tired? Have you lost weight?"*
   - obtained important information about the patient's family history, which led to a deeper understanding of her concerns
   - obtained information about her feelings regarding her work as a dental nurse, which may account for her irritability – dissatisfaction with work is noted as a differential diagnosis but is not offered to the patient as a possibility on this occasion
   - explored the patient's health understanding by asking *"what made you suspect diabetes?"*
   - explored the patient's concerns: *"What's raising your concerns?"*
   - explored the patient's expectations: *"Would you like to talk to Dr Brown? Are you happy for me to have a quiet word with Dr Brown?"*

2. *Performs an appropriate physical or mental examination*
   - The patient was questioned about sleep, tiredness and weight loss, which are also depressive symptoms.

   The doctor could have:
   - formally assessed BP and weight

B. Clinical management skills

3. *Make an appropriate working diagnosis*
   - The doctor made a working diagnosis of a dissatisfied patient who may have diabetes mellitus.
   - The case was written as an angry patient who threatens to complain. Not all her symptoms suggest diabetes and there is some doubt about the likelihood of this diagnosis.

4. *Explain the problem to the patient using appropriate language*
   The doctor could have:
   - provided more in the way of explanation of each problem

5. *Provide holistic care and use resources effectively*
The doctor:
- was informed by guidelines: http://cks.library.nhs.uk/diabetes_glycaemic_control/making_a_diagnosis and www.nhs.uk/chq/Pages/1083.aspx?CategoryID=68&SubCategoryID=162
- tackled both issues and so provided holistic care; the doctor created a reasonable relationship with the patient to enable on-going care
- made cost-effective use of resources by requesting a fasting blood glucose rather than a GTT

6. *Prescribe appropriately*
- The doctor did not prescribe, which was appropriate in this case.

7. *Specify the conditions and interval for follow-up*
The doctor:
- arranged a fasting blood test

The doctor could have:
- specified a time-scale for the bloods and arranged a follow-up appointment to review the results

C. Interpersonal skills: know and treat this patient

8. *Achieve rapport*
The doctor:
- actively listened and summarised
- regularly checked understanding – in doing so, she refrained from offering superfluous advice on how to formalise a complaint and potential lifestyle changes
- chose not to challenge an angry patient on their first meeting and concentrated instead on establishing a cordial professional relationship
- explored the patient's concerns about early diabetes and addressed her expectations for better testing

9. *Give the patient the opportunity to be involved in significant management decisions*
The doctor:
- offered ways in which the patient could act on her feelings towards Dr Brown

The doctor could have:
- discussed the different diagnostic tests for diabetes and offered the patient a choice; however, this needs to be balanced against risking a longer consultation and justifying the cost of a GGT

Debrief

What could you learn from this consultation? How to
- summarise – to indicate active listening and to structure the consultation
- obtain a psycho-social history
- explore the patient's ideas, concerns and expectations
- be non-judgemental
- deal with two important issues within ten minutes

Summary of learning

Write your answers in the space provided.

1. What questions would you ask to explore the differential diagnosis?

2. What would you say to the patient to involve her in the management plan?

3. How could you specify review or follow-up?

4. If the patient were unaware of the complaints procedure, how would you explain it to her?

Relevant literature

Jain A, Ogden J (1999) A qualitative study of general practitioners' experiences of a patient complaint. *BMJ*; **318**: 1596–1599 (www.bmj.com/cgi/content/abstract/318/7198/1596)

http://cks.library.nhs.uk/diabetes_glycaemic_control/making_a_diagnosis

www.nhs.uk/chq/Pages/1083.aspx?CategoryID=68&SubCategoryID=162

Video 3 - Pregnant and worried

Brief to the doctor

Mrs GP is a 28 year old woman who has recently registered with your practice. She is pregnant and has seen the midwife for two routine checks.

Patient summary

Name   GP

Date of birth (Age)   28

Social and Family History   Married, 1st pregnancy

Past medical history   Eczema

Repeat medication   Diprobase as directed

Tasks for the doctor when watching the case

The tasks are to:
- notice how the doctor barely spoke at the start of the consultation – this allowed the patient to air her fears and get her concerns off her chest – which in a consultation about social or emotional issues can be therapeutic in itself
- notice how the doctor summarised the patient's presenting problem and highlighted three main issues; the overt structure enabled systematic questioning and explanation
- notice how the doctor interrupted the patient at several points, without annoying the patient. The interruptions occurred at points in the consultation when the patient repeated herself. The interruptions redirected the patient to the main issues. The doctor was able to gather, in the time provided, sufficient data to explore the reasons for the patient's fears and to 'objectively' assess her risk of harm.
- see how the doctor identified the benefits of the patient disclosing her fears to her husband. The patient felt unable to initiate the conversation with her husband, but the doctor suggested a strategy to overcome this barrier, thereby moving the consultation forward.
- notice that, although a good therapeutic relationship was established and follow-up offered, alternative sources of support, such as the midwife, were not suggested
- comment on the doctor's decision to neither prescribe nor refer
- comment on whether sufficient information about the patient's support network or the husband's job stresses was obtained to inform the risk assessment

Review of the doctor's approach

A. Data gathering, examination and clinical assessment skills

1. *Define the clinical problem: clarify why the patient has presented today*
   The doctor:
   - established good rapport by actively listening and by using the patient's words and terminology in questioning and explanations
   - reflected and summarised the history
   - made systematic enquiries along three defined strands
   - asked open questions to explore the problem, such as *"what makes you think he is distant? What do you think is causing that distance? What makes you think he is not interested in the baby?"*
   - asked closed questions to assess the likelihood of harm to the patient: *"did he ask you to have a termination? Did he come with you to the scans? He hasn't got a history of violence, has he?"*
   - obtained information about the husband's occupation; however, the cue about him being in the military was not followed up by questions about the patient's social support (such as whether she is living away from family) or the husband's work pressures
   - obtained important 'red flag' information about her husband's character, whether he was aggressive or had a history of violence, but alcohol or drug use was not queried
   - uncovered the patient's concern about her husband's attitude potentially affecting the baby and explored the reasons for that concern, i.e. the newspaper article about a man who fed his partner 'abortion' pills and killed her baby
   - satisfied the patient's stated expectation (*"I've come for a chat"*). The chat served two purposes: first, it helped the patient to make sense of her feelings, and, secondly, the doctor made offers of help. Hence, the patient was empowered to deal with the problem.

2. *Performs an appropriate physical or mental examination*
   - An examination was not undertaken.

B. Clinical management skills

3. *Make an appropriate working diagnosis*
   - The doctor made a working diagnosis of there being a difference between the expectation and reality of the husband's feelings and behaviours towards the pregnancy, however, this was not pathological.
   - The case was written as about an expectant mum who, after reading a newspaper article about a man who fed his partner 'abortion pills', works herself up into an almost irrational fear for her baby. The doctor needed

to assess her risk of harm. If the risk was assessed incorrectly, the doctor may have made unnecessary referrals or prescribed inappropriately. If the doctor failed to 'listen' to the patient's concerns, she would have felt patronised and become tearful.

4. *Explain the problem to the patient using appropriate language*
   - The doctor spoke about there being a spectrum of reactions to fatherhood. While everyday language was used, the word 'horrible' failed to convey the same meaning as 'pathological'. Perhaps the word 'criminal' would have been more appropriate.

5. *Provide holistic care and use resources effectively*
   The doctor:
   - dealt with a social and emotional issue in a sensitive and constructive manner, hence holistic care was provided. The doctor created a reasonable relationship with the patient to enable on-going care.

   However, the doctor did not:
   - signpost to alternative sources of support, such as the midwife or local volunteer agencies; in the military, the padre also provides pastoral support and counselling

6. *Prescribe appropriately*
   - The doctor did not prescribe, which was appropriate in this case.

7. *Specify the conditions and interval for follow-up*
   - The doctor and patient agreed to meet again if needed.

C. Interpersonal skills: know and treat this patient

8. *Achieve rapport*
   The doctor:
   - actively listened and summarised: *"it seems to me that ..."*
   - checked agreement at several points: *"do you feel happy to have that conversation?"*
   - understood the patient's reaction to the newspaper article; by being supportive, empathetic but detached, the doctor helped the patient to achieve insight and perspective

9. *Give the patient the opportunity to be involved in significant management decisions*
   - The doctor made offers: *"do you feel happy to have that conversation? Do you think you would be able to take this first step more easily now?"*

Debrief

What could you learn from this consultation? How to
- reflect and summarise, using the phrase: *"it seems to me ..."*
- move the consultation forward: after gathering the relevant data, formulate a management plan that empowers the patient
- make offers and check agreement
- deal with challenging social and emotional issues within ten minutes

Summary of learning

Write your answers in the space provided.

1. What questions would you ask to assess the patient's risk of harm from her husband?

2. How would you explain the problem to the patient using words she is likely to understand?

3. What would your management plan be? How would you explain the plan to the patient?

4. If the patient was socially isolated (living away from family and had not made friends at the military base) and her husband had a history of alcohol binge drinking, would your management change? Justify your decision.

Relevant literature

For the original article read by the patient, follow *The Guardian* link: http://lifeandhealth.guardian.co.uk/women/story/0,,2270135,00.html

This was a challenging consultation about a social and emotional issue. If the doctor felt overwhelmed by the patient's presentation, one approach would be to structure the consultation using a consultation model. In this case, the Calgary–Cambridge approach was used. To revise consultation models, see: www.skillscascade.com/models.htm

Video 4 – Repeat script and husband snores

Brief to the doctor

Mrs PB is a 42 year old woman who presents with two problems: first, she requests a repeat prescription of her contraceptive pill, and secondly, she wants to explore what can be done to help her husband's snoring.

Patient summary

Name   PB

Date of birth (Age)   42

Past medical history   Non-focal migraine on combined oral contraception

Repeat medication   Cerazette, one tablet daily × 126

Tasks for the doctor when watching the case

The tasks are to:
- take note of how the doctor explored both agendas within the allocated time
- notice how the doctor gathered sufficient data to prescribe safely
- observe how the doctor communicated the risks and benefits of the Mirena intra-uterine system (IUS) in a way that was meaningful to the patient
- comment on the doctor's non-verbal communication: posture, use of hands, facial expressions
- assess whether the patient felt empowered by the advice she was given on treatments for snoring
- evaluate whether the patient was given the opportunity to be involved in the management plan

Review of the doctor's approach

A. Data gathering, examination and clinical assessment skills

1. Define the clinical problem: clarify why the patient has presented today
The doctor:
- made good eye contact, nodded appropriately, and encouraged the patient to talk; however, questions such as *"is that what you wanted to talk about today?"* and *"is that alright?"* discouraged a deeper exploration of the main issue, namely marital strain to which snoring was one of many contributing factors.
- asked open questions to explore the problem, such as *"how are you getting on with [cerazette]?"* and *"how about the migraine side of things?"*
- asked closed questions to clarify details about the snoring: *"is this placing a strain on your relationship? Have you discussed this with him?"*

The doctor could have:
- gained more information about how the snoring affected the patient and her marital relationship by asking neutral questions. When the doctor attempted to explore the patient's irritability and grumpiness, he attributed her feelings to a low mood, and the patient corrected him by saying her feelings were due to her husband's snoring rather than an intrinsic mood disorder. The patient may have felt that the doctor was jumping to the wrong conclusions and consequently may not have felt that the doctor had truly listened to her concerns.
- explored the patient's health understanding by asking about what had led her to believe that an operation for her husband's snoring would be the solution to their marriage difficulties. The doctor did not respond to the verbal cue: *"you hear about ops"*
- identified and addressed the patient's frustrations with not being able to persuade her husband to seek help. It seemed that she was canvassing the doctor for written information about snoring treatments but these expectations were neither acknowledged nor met.

2. Performs an appropriate physical or mental examination
An examination was not essential.

B. Clinical management skills

3. Make an appropriate working diagnosis
- The doctor made a working diagnosis of 'safe to repeat the prescription for the progestogen-only pill (POP), and husband snores, probably due to recent weight gain'.
- The case was written about the hidden agenda, with the marital difficulties being the real reason for the consultation. The patient, at several points

during the consultation, stressed that she was happy with her Pill. She pulled a face when alternative contraception was discussed, a cue that this was not her primary concern. However, when talking about her husband's snoring, she volunteered information about a *"recent fight"* and described her frustration with her inability to find a solution to the problem of his snoring. She was stuck and wanted help with the snoring problem.

4. *Explain the problem to the patient using appropriate language*
The doctor:
- explored whether the POP was a reasonable and safe contraceptive choice prior to prescribing
- offered long-acting contraception alternatives, in line with NICE guidance
- offered to see the patient's husband and volunteered information on treatments for snoring, namely weight reduction and operations on the palate

However, the doctor:
- used words such as 'palate' and 'oestrogen' without explanation and the assessor is not sure if the language used was 'appropriate' to the patient's understanding. The patient, having already asked if it was OK to broach the subject of her husband's snoring (*"do we have time to talk about another issue?"*), may not have volunteered her lack of understanding.
- in prescribing the POP, did not demonstrate an attempt to enhance concordance

5. *Provide holistic care and use resources effectively*
The doctor:
- addressed both issues (contraception and snoring)
- was informed by guidelines:
  www.nice.org.uk/guidance/index.jsp?action=byID&o=10974

However, the assessor is unsure if:
- holistic care was provided: the issue of snoring was superficially explored, and so it was difficult to move the problem forward. Had the doctor uncovered the patient's true concerns and expectations, the doctor could have designed a more inclusive and holistic management plan.
- the patient left the consultation armed with new information that could persuade her husband to see his GP. Hence marks cannot be awarded for 'empowering the patient'.

6. *Prescribe appropriately*
The doctor could have:
- checked the patient's understanding of the amounts of medication required and asked if she had a family planning booklet for written advice on 'missed pills' and commonly occurring pill interactions

7. *Specify the conditions and interval for follow-up*
The doctor could have:
- signposted the patient to information on treatments for snoring or given a leaflet detailing the medical help available
- specified when he would like to review the patient again, such as by saying *"I have given you a prescription for a six month supply of the Pill. Please see me or the practice nurse for a review in six months".*

C. Interpersonal skills: know and treat this patient

8. *Achieve rapport*
The doctor:
- listened attentively to the patient's description of her two presenting problems
- reflected appropriately: *"is this putting a strain on your relationship?"*
- asked if there was anything further the patient required at the end of the consultation: *"is that alright?"*

9. *Give the patient the opportunity to be involved in significant management decisions*
The doctor could have:
- encouraged the patient's involvement in the management plan: *"I have suggested your husband come and see us for weight loss advice and for further information on operations for snoring. What do you think about this plan?"*

Debrief

- What could you learn from this consultation? How to
  - take a systematic and focused history for safe POP prescribing
  - address two issues in 10 minutes
  - be efficient with time (by avoiding unnecessary examinations)
- What questions could you ask to discover the patient's concerns and expectations?
- How would you explore the issue of the husband's snoring?
- How could you briefly outline long-acting contraceptive alternatives to the patient?
- How could you involve the patient in the management plan?

Relevant literature

For an excellent overview of various contraceptive choices, see www.youtube.com – search for 'Contraception Owens' for a video-clip by Annette Owens.

For information on long-acting contraception, see www.nice.org.uk/guidance/index. jsp?action=byID&o=10974.

For an overview of initial treatments for snoring see www.youtube.com – search for 'snoring + advice' for a video-clip from a Good Morning Texas broadcast.

Video 5 – Infertility

Brief to the doctor

Mrs CD is a 28 year old woman who presents with difficulty in conceiving.

Patient summary

Name	CD
Date of birth (Age)	28
Past medical history	Nil of significance
Repeat medication	None for the last year

Tasks for the doctor when watching the case

The tasks are to:
- take note of the 'wait time', that is the length of the pause, or the time taken for the doctor to make the shift from listening to the patient to questioning her (for a detailed explanation of 'wait time', see www.commscascade.medschl.cam.ac.uk/pages/whatteach.html and click on 'attentive listening' under Specific Skills).
- comment on how the doctor signalled to the patient to continue telling her story. Look at the use of head nods, facial expression and neutral facilitative comments such as *"uh-huh"*, *"right"* and *"I see"*.
- assess the doctor's tone, rate and volume of speech and comment on its impact on the consultation
- comment on the doctor's ability to phrase and deliver information about investigation for infertility in a way the patient was able to understand
- assess whether the information given was needed or wanted
- assess whether the doctor checked to see how the patient was reacting to what she said?

Review of the doctor's approach

A. Data gathering, examination and clinical assessment skills

1. *Define the clinical problem: clarify why the patient has presented today*
   The doctor:
   - invited the patient into the room, smiled warmly, sat facing the patient, nodded appropriately, and paused after the patient spoke thereby signalling a willingness to listen and encouraging the patient to tell her story
   - asked reflective questions, using the patient's words and phrasing, such as *"some time?"* and *"when you thought of a referral?"*
   - after establishing the reason for the patient's attendance, progressed to the data gathering section of the consultation using sign-posting and transitional statements, such as *"I don't know you. I'm going to ask you quite a few questions to see how I can best help you."* The transfer from an open to closed style of questioning was made clear to the patient – signposted. As this was done explicitly, the patient was not disturbed by the change in questioning style.
   - asked closed questions to clarify details about the gynaecological history: *"do you have gynae problems? Pelvic infection? Pelvic or abdominal surgery?"*
   - explored the patient's expectations by asking *"when you came in, what were you hoping to get from this consultation? When you thought of a referral, were there any tests you had in mind?"*
   - explored the patient's concerns: *"how do you feel about [the guidelines for referral in the UK being different to the Australian guidance]?"*

   The doctor could have:
   - gained more social and psychological information such as whether the patient came from a large family or whether there was any expectation from her husband or family for her to become pregnant quickly

2. *Performs an appropriate physical or mental examination*
   - Prior to requesting blood tests, the doctor checked for pallor. The examination was targeted, that is, if pallor was noted, it would be appropriate to request a FBC

   The doctor could have:
   - taken her BP

B. Clinical management skills

3. *Make an appropriate working diagnosis*
   - The doctor made a working diagnosis of 'difficulty conceiving; no indication for early fertility clinic referral in a woman under 35 years'.
   - The case was written to be difficulty conceiving, in a well-informed health care worker (pharmacist) who has read widely around the topic on the internet.

4. *Explain the problem to the patient using appropriate language*
   The doctor:
   - explained the UK fertility referral guidelines to the patient using reassuring statements and humour
   - provided the correct amount and type of information
   - involved the patient – shared thinking, explained rationale, explained why some blood tests (and not others) were requested

5. *Provide holistic care and use resources effectively*
   The doctor:
   - was informed by guidelines (http://cks.library.nhs.uk/infertility#-296878)
   - provided holistic care by addressing issues such as regular sexual intercourse, folic acid intake, cervical smears, and lifestyle
   - used resources effectively, requesting appropriate and targeted blood tests

   However, chlamydia screening was not discussed.

6. *Prescribe appropriately*
   The doctor:
   - appropriately chose not to prescribe

7. *Specify the conditions and interval for follow-up*
   The doctor:
   - advised the patient to make an appointment for non-fasting blood tests

   The doctor could have:
   - arranged for chlamydia screening for both partners
   - offered to see the husband for a general health check and consultation
   - arranged for semen analysis

C. Interpersonal skills: know and treat this patient

8. *Achieve rapport*
   The doctor:
   - used 'wait time' effectively – her pauses gave the patient time to think, to contribute more, and to speak for longer; the doctor needed to ask fewer questions to extract the important information
   - spoke slowly, looked interested and made good eye contact signalling her interest in the patient's problem and her willingness to help

9. *Give the patient the opportunity to be involved in significant management decisions*
   The doctor:
   - encouraged autonomy by asking the patient if blood tests were something she'd be interested in; she involved the patient in the management plan

Debrief

- What could you learn from this consultation? How to:
  - take an accurate, systematic and focused clinical history
  - weave in the patient's framework
  - build the relationship with the patient
  - explain, give information and plan without repetition
  - devise a joint management plan that is acceptable to the patient
- How would you negotiate the decision not to refer with the patient?
- How would you encourage the patient to persuade her husband to attend?

Relevant literature

For an excellent website on consultation skills, see www.commscascade.medschl.cam.ac.uk/

For information on infertility, see www.emedicine.com/med/topic3535.htm

Video 6 – Domestic violence

Brief to the doctor

Miss SB is a 23 year old woman who has recently moved to the local area after her partner was posted on to the neighbouring military base. Her notes have not arrived as yet. This is her first consultation and she presents with domestic violence.

Patient summary

The medical record has not arrived into your practice as yet.

Tasks for the doctor when watching the case

The tasks are to:
- evaluate how the doctor enabled and encouraged the doctor–patient partnership
- notice how the doctor promoted openness and trust to facilitate mutual decision-making
- comment on the doctor's decision not to exchange information with outside agencies
- assess whether the doctor responded flexibly to the patient's expectations and needs
- evaluate whether the doctor created a therapeutic relationship in which the patient could be supported over a period of time

Review of the doctor's approach

A. Data gathering, examination and clinical assessment skills

1. *Define the clinical problem: clarify why the patient has presented today*
   The doctor:
   - demonstrated acceptance, that is, she accepted non-judgementally what the patient said. By accepting the patients' ideas and emotions without initially interrogating or dissuading her, she acknowledged the patient's position and feelings.
   - demonstrated empathy; this was achieved in several ways: she matched her tone of voice to the patient's, she did less of the talking, and she refrained from dispensing advice
   - picked up on the patient's confusion over who was to blame for the violence, tentatively explored the issue, and then reassured with sensitivity

- asked open questions to explore the problem, such as *"what is the situation at the moment?"* and *"what violence has there been?"*
- asked closed questions to clarify details about the domestic violence: *"was that a significant injury? Do you have any children? Are you financially dependent on him? Have you spoken to him?"*
- explored the patient's ideas: *"Are you feeling as if it's your fault?"*
- explored the patient's concerns by asking *"what will happen if you stay?"*
- explored the patient's expectations: *"would you like me to refer you to somebody? What about a drop-in centre?"*

The doctor could have:

- gained more information on the patient's support network, such as the physical distance away from family and friends, and whether her partner also frightened them – this is important should she require refuge from her current living situation
- asked about the partner's alcohol or drug use, and whether or not he had a criminal record

2. *Performs an appropriate physical or mental examination*
   - A formal examination was not required.

B. Clinical management skills

3. *Make an appropriate working diagnosis*
   - The doctor made a working diagnosis of 'domestic violence, mainly emotional and psychological but also physical'
   - The case was written to be domestic violence in a young socially isolated woman who is beginning to believe that she is somehow to blame and who is uncertain about leaving because of economic and emotional repercussions.

4. *Explain the problem to the patient using appropriate language*
   The doctor:
   - explained that abused women are often made to feel that they are somehow to blame
   - gave an explanation that was concise and understandable
   - did not give advice or reassure prematurely

5. *Provide holistic care and use resources effectively*
   The doctor:
   - was informed by guidelines (RCGP, Domestic violence: the general practitioner's role: www.rcgp.org.uk/Default.aspx?page=2259)
   - encouraged the patient to contribute her preferences for treatment by asking: *"what would you like to do about this?"*
   - involved the patient by making suggestions (about referrals, involving outside agencies or looking on the internet) rather than directing the

patient to what the doctor thought was best. By offering choices, a mutually acceptable plan was negotiated. Had the initial plan (of referral) not been checked with the patient, the barriers to successful treatment (boyfriend checking mail and texts) would not have been addressed.

- safety netted by offering her realistic choices for follow-up while accepting that the decisions regarding treatment were hers alone

However, the assessor is unsure if:

- the patient was offered help in contacting any of the suggested agencies, such as the local women's aid refuge, local authority social services department, or the Department of Social Security
- the patient was advised on how to plan for an emergency, of a financial or personal safety nature

6. *Prescribe appropriately*
- The doctor, appropriately, did not prescribe.

7. *Specify the conditions and interval for follow-up*
The doctor:
- signposted the patient to appropriate information
- suggested to the patient that she would like to *"meet up"* again – it was more appropriate to make an offer than to contract follow up

C. Interpersonal skills: know and treat this patient

8. *Achieve rapport*
The doctor:
- was not judgemental
- communicated her understanding and appreciation of the patient's predicament (*"if he doesn't know what will make him happy, how could you know?"*)
- provided support: expressed concern, understanding and willingness to help (*"This sounds like an awful situation. You don't sound very hopeful"*)
- dealt sensitively with a disturbing topic

9. *Give the patient the opportunity to be involved in significant management decisions*
The doctor:
- shared thinking with the patient to encourage her involvement (*"it seems to me that you are in the process of exploring your options"*)
- offered options – her efforts were directed towards enabling the patient to make the decisions best suited to her personal circumstances

Debrief

- What could you learn from this consultation? How to:
  - discuss a difficult topic with sensitivity
  - support the patient
  - tactfully offer an opinion of what is going on
  - be efficient with time
- What questions could you ask to explore what support she has available from family and friends?
- If she had a bruise on her hand, would you examine her? To what extent?
- How could you explain the rationale and purpose of your examination to her?
- If she disclosed that she was concerned about the safety of her child, how would your management plan change? What would you say to her?

Relevant literature

Dr Iona Heath (RCGP) *Domestic violence: the general practitioner's role*, available on-line: www.rcgp.org.uk/Default.aspx?page=2259

For information on acceptance and empathy, see:
www.gp-training.net/training/communication_skills/calgary/rapport.htm

Video 7 – Chest pain

Brief to the doctor

Ms TR is a 60 year old woman who presents with chest pain. She has registered as a temporary patient. She lives in Austria and is visiting her grandchildren in the UK. She wants to know if she is fit to fly to Austria tomorrow.

Patient summary

Name	TR
Date of birth (Age)	60
Past medical history	None recorded
Repeat medication	None recorded

Tasks for the doctor when watching the case

The tasks are to:

- take note of how the doctor assessed the patient's ideas, concerns and expectations within the opening minutes of the consultation
- notice how the doctor signposted the patient to the history taking, warning her that she was about to ask several questions about the condition and risk factors for heart disease
- comment on the choice of the doctor's examination – she took the pulse, BP, auscultated the heart and examined the neck veins. Would you have done a more or less detailed examination? What would you examine and why?
- did the patient appear to understand the explanation? If yes, what made the explanation easy to understand? If no, what would you do to improve the explanation? What words would you use?
- Notice how the doctor safety-netted (GTN prescription and letter to Austrian GP). Do you think this is adequate? Should the doctor have advised the patient to warn the airline or ask for oxygen?
- Would you have requested a baseline ECG or a pin-prick haemoglobin? Justify your answer.

Review of the doctor's approach

A. Data gathering, examination and clinical assessment skills

1. *Define the clinical problem: clarify why the patient has presented today*
   The doctor:
   - hardly spoke during the 'Golden Minute' – she simply facilitated disclosure in the 1st minute by nodding her head and saying *"right"*
   - responded to the patient's cue with *"you look a bit worried"*
   - elicited the patient's concerns: *"What are you hoping this won't be?"*
   - signposted the patient to the raft of open and closed questions she was about to ask about the chest pain and risk factors for heart disease
   - used explorative questions such as *"what happens at the top of the hill?"* and *"what made you give up [smoking]?"*
   - used closed questions to clarify details: *"How many times did you get pain? Do you suffer from hypertension?"*
   - prefaced the examination by saying *"there's still a bit we don't know. Let's examine you first..."*

   The doctor could have:
   - gained more psycho-social information about how the patient was *"coping with all this? Is it having an effect on the visit?"*
   - asked whether the patient was concerned about flying with the pain. Did the patient want to know if she should inform the airline or change her travel arrangements?

2. *Performs an appropriate physical or mental examination*
   - The pulse, BP, chest and neck veins were examined; hence the examination was appropriate and directed.
   - The doctor said to the patient *"you have a fantastic BP. Is that due to exercise?"*

   According to Sign Guidance (2001):
   - weight, height, body mass index, and waist circumference should be measured
   - evidence of hyperlipidaemia (e.g. xanthelasma, tendon xanthomata), vascular disease (e.g. absent foot pulses, bruits) anaemia or hyperthyroidism should be sought

   For fitness to fly with stable angina, the patient should not have a Hb <7.5 g/dl.

   What examinations would you do? Comment on the fluency of your technique.

B. Clinical management skills

3. *Make an appropriate working diagnosis*
   - Prior to launching into an explanation, the doctor asked *"what do you know about angina?"*.
   - The doctor explained angina simply using language – pictures or leaflets were not used.
   - The case was written to be the initial presentation of stable angina in a temporary resident who is needs an urgent assessment of fitness to fly. The doctor has to decide which examination and investigations need to be undertaken urgently to inform the risk assessment for fitness to fly. Decisions regarding travel and medication need to be made in the face of uncertainty.

4. *Explain the problem to the patient using appropriate language*
   The doctor:
   - attempted to explain the diagnosis to the patient using phrases such as *"furring of the blood vessels"* and *"increased work of the heart"*
   - prescribed GTN spray appropriately (the British Airways website advises that patients with angina may fly and asks them to remember to carry their medication on their person).

5. *Provide holistic care and use resources effectively*
   The doctor:
   - was informed by guidelines (www.sign.ac.uk/pdf/sign96.pdf)
   - provided holistic care: the issue of fitness to fly was addressed and the patient was asked *"how do you feel about flying tomorrow?"*
   - used resources effectively: the doctor offered to post a letter to the patient or her GP, outlining the discussion today and leaving future investigations (blood tests and stress ECG) up to the clinician with overall responsibility for the patient's care

   However, the assessor is unsure:
   - if sufficient data were gathered (emotional precipitants for chest pain, anaemia and exclusion of baseline ECG changes) to inform a through risk assessment. The case was written such that if the doctor asked for a baseline ECG, the patient would have handed over a copy of the ECG saying the triage nurse *"thought you may want this"*.

6. *Prescribe appropriately*
   The doctor:
   - prescribed GTN spray as an interim measure should anything happen on the flight
   - asked *"do you know about GTN sprays"*

7. *Specify the conditions and interval for follow-up*
The doctor:

- advised the patient to see her GP to organise further investigation

However, the assessor is unsure that:

- the patient understood the time-scale in which this should be done

C. Interpersonal skills: know and treat this patient

8. *Achieve rapport*
The doctor:

- listened attentively to the patient's description of her problem
- recognised the patient's concern that she may have a heart problem
- asked if she had answered her queries about medication, flying and ability to organise further tests through her GP in Austria

9. *Give the patient the opportunity to be involved in significant management decisions*
The doctor:

- encouraged autonomy by asking whether the patient felt more comfortable taking or not taking the GTN spray on to the flight. Had the patient said she was uncomfortable, then the reasons for this could have been explored and addressed.

Debrief

- What could you learn from this consultation? How to:
  - ○ facilitate information gathering in the 'Golden Minute'
  - ○ signpost prior to taking a systematic and focused history
  - ○ decide which examinations to perform to inform your risk assessment
  - ○ explain conditions in simple language, avoiding jargon
  - ○ be efficient with resources
- How would you assess the patient's fitness to fly?
- How would you examine the cardiovascular system?
- How would you involve the patient in the management plan?

Relevant literature

For an excellent website detailing the examination of the heart, with links to heart sounds, see: http://meded.ucsd.edu/clinicalmed/heart.htm

For information on fitness to fly with medical conditions, see www.ba.com then click on 'Information', and then on 'Medical Information' under the 'Travel Preparation' tab and http://whqlibdoc.who.int/publications/2005/9241580364_chap2.pdf

For a useful consultation guide, see
www.pennine-gp-training.co.uk/Useful-phrases-for-achieving--COT-competencies.doc

Video 8 – Pregnancy

Brief to the doctor

Mrs PB is a 34 year old woman who presents with a positive pregnancy test. She wants to know about maternity benefits.

Patient summary

Name	PB
Date of birth (Age)	34
Past medical history	6 week postnatal check completed (19 February)
	Vaginal delivery with episiotomy (10 January)
Current medication	Diclofenac 50 mg thrice daily × 42T (10 January)
Blood tests	Tests were done 3 weeks ago
Hb	11.2 g/dl (12–15)
MCV	99 (83–105)
White cell count	7.32 (4–11)
Differential count	no abnormalities
Platelet count	354 (150–400)

Tasks for the doctor

Read the NICE guidance on antenatal care at: www.nice.org.uk/guidance/index.jsp?action=byID&o=11947 or go to www.nice.org.uk/ and search for Antenatal Care

NICE advises that a pregnant woman, at the first contact with a healthcare professional, receives:
- folic acid supplementation
- advice on food hygiene, including how to reduce the risk of a food-acquired infection
- lifestyle advice, including smoking cessation, and the implications of recreational drug use and alcohol consumption in pregnancy
- advice on all antenatal screening, including screening for haemoglobinopathies, the anomaly scan and screening for Down syndrome, as well as risks and benefits of the screening tests

For guidance on Statutory Maternity Pay (SMP), see: www.pensionsadvisoryservice.org.uk/workplace-pension-schemes/final-salary-schemes/maternity-leave.

SMP is paid for 39 weeks. In this case, the doctor needs to ascertain when the current maternity leave started and count 39 weeks to determine when it runs out. The case was written for maternity leave to have started on 2 January. Therefore, SMP ends in October.

The earliest date that new SMP can start is from the 11th week before the week the baby is due. In this case, if the EDD for the current pregnancy is 5 November, then SMP may start at the end of August. The patient can be advised to start her new SMP when her current SMP ends.

www.dwp.gov.uk/advisers/ni17a/smp/smp_2.asp:
To qualify for SMP, the patient must be in continuous employment, usually employment by the same employer without a break, except under some circumstances when employment can be treated as continuous in spite of some breaks, such as absence (for periods of 26 consecutive weeks or less) because of sickness, injury, pregnancy or childbirth.

Having read the above guidance, watch case 8 on the DVD. Mark the candidate according to the schedule listed below.

Generic indicators for targeted assessment domains	Descriptors – positive and negative
A. Data gathering, technical and assessment skills • Gathering of data for clinical judgement, choice of examination, investigations and their interpretations • Demonstrating proficiency in performing physical examinations and using diagnostic and therapeutic instruments Maps on the blueprint to: • **Data gathering and interpretation (A)** • **Technical skills (F)**	Positive indicators: • correctly establishes the EDD • takes a focused obstetric history, establishing the need for folic acid supplementation and iron treatment • elicits what the patient already knows about antenatal care and screening • finds out when current maternity leave commenced, or signposts to resources with information on SMP Negative indicators: • is unable to calculate the EDD • does not identify need for folic acid and iron treatment • appears disorganised or unsystematic in taking a relevant gynaecological and obstetric history • fails to identify when current SMP ends and date from which new SMP can be claimed, or fails to signpost to resources to provide this information

B. Clinical management skills	Positive indicators:
• Recognition and management of common medical conditions in primary care. Demonstrates flexible and structured approach to decision making. • Demonstrating ability to deal with multiple complaints and co-morbidity and to promote a shared approach to managing problems Maps on the blueprint to: • **Management (B)** • **Co-morbidity and health promotion (C)**	• clarifies for patient the date of expected delivery and end of first trimester • discusses routine ANC • prescribes the correct dose of folic acid and ferrous sulphate and takes steps to improve concordance • refers appropriately to the midwife Negative indicators: • fails to clarify for patient the date of expected delivery and end of first trimester • fails to discuss routine ANC • fails to prescribe the correct dose of folic acid and ferrous sulphate and/or fails to improve concordance • fails to refer to the midwife or refers inappropriately to resources for high-risk pregnancies
C. Interpersonal skills	Positive indicators:
• Use of recognised communication techniques that enhance understanding of a patient's illness and promote a shared approach to managing problems • Practising ethically with respect for equality and diversity in line with accepted codes of professional conduct Maps on the blueprint to: • **Person-centred approach (D)** • **Professional attitude (E)**	• shows empathy to the patient's embarrassment and takes steps to put her at ease • involves the patient in the management plan • addresses the patient's expectations regarding SMP and her queries regarding what she should tell her employers Negative indicators: • fails to put the patient at ease or embarrasses her further • fails to involve the patient in the management plan; gives formulaic ANC advice and prescriptions • fails to acknowledge the patient's expectations regarding SMP and employment

Debrief

- What could you learn from this consultation? How to:
  - establish rapport, show empathy and put the patient at ease
  - explore the patient's health understanding regarding ANC so as not to repeat advice
  - take steps to enhance concordance
  - be efficient with time
- How would you focus and structure the history taking?
- What ANC advice would you provide?
- What prescriptions would you write?
- How would you deal with the request for information on SMP and returning to work?

Relevant literature

www.nice.org.uk/guidance/index.jsp?action=byID&o=11947 or go to www.nice.org.uk/ and search for Antenatal Care.

For information on SMP, see www.dwp.gov.uk and search for SMP.

Video 9 – Pre-wedding diet pills

Brief to the doctor

Miss LA is a 28 year old woman who presents with an internet printout on a 'diet patch'. She wants to know about the efficacy and safety of the patch.

Patient summary

Name	LA
Date of birth (Age)	28
Past medical history	Low back pain (2 months ago) – referred to physiotherapy
Current medication	Ibuprofen 400 mg thrice daily × 84T (2 months ago)

Tasks for the doctor

This case is written to test how well the candidate consults with a woman presenting with an internet printout. The case is weighted to assess the doctor's interpersonal skills, that is, his ability to consult in a patient-centred manner.

Read the information provided on the advantages and disadvantages of internet printouts, guidance on how to deal with the situation and the characteristics of patient-centred consulting. Then watch the DVD and mark the case.

For information on the pros and cons of internet printouts, see: www.jmir.org/2002/1/e5/. Poor quality information may result in misdiagnosis and mistreatment. However, the advantages are:
- increased information – with improved understanding and self-care
- reduction in clinician consultations
- prompt help-seeking when needed
- a medium for social support, by providing patients with narratives about another's experience of illness. Texts written by patients may provide the personal experience and reassurance desired.

For guidance on how to deal with the internet printouts, see Brown (2003) article in *Pulse*. When a patient presents with an internet printout, try to determine the patient's agenda.
- Why did they do this? What specific questions did they have?
- Are they unhappy with their current management?

- Did they find this exercise useful? If so why?
- Have they had previous experience with online searching?

What should the doctor do?
- Remember patients are asking for the doctor's advice and opinion, probably because they value it.
- Once doctors have elucidated the patient's concerns, questions and anxieties, appraise the information.
- Cross-check with reference sources such as textbooks.
- Discuss the findings.

For the characteristics of patient-centred consulting, see Little *et al.* (2001) in the *BMJ*. Patient-centred care is care which:
- explores the patient's main reason for the visit, concerns, and need for information
- seeks an integrated understanding of the patient's world – that is, their whole person, emotional needs, and life issues
- finds common ground on what the problem is and mutually agrees on management; enhances prevention and health promotion
- enhances the continuing relationship between the patient and the doctor

Having read the above guidance, watch case 9 on the DVD. Mark the candidate according to the schedule listed below.

Generic indicators for targeted assessment domains	Descriptors – positive and negative
A. Data gathering, technical and assessment skills • Gathering of data for clinical judgement, choice of examination, investigations and their interpretations • Demonstrating proficiency in performing physical examinations and using diagnostic and therapeutic instruments Maps on the blueprint to: • **Data gathering and interpretation (A)** • **Technical skills (F)**	Positive indicators: • correctly establishes why the patient presents – for help in appraising the safety and efficacy of the diet patch • elicits why the patient looked for information on the internet • uncovers the patient's concern about her appearance in her wedding dress and in swimwear • finds out what measures the patient has already tried and whether these have been successful Negative indicators: • is bewildered by the information presented; assumes the patient is requesting prescription diet pills • does not identify the patient's wants and needs • does not identify the patient's ideas (herbal is safe), concerns (fat tummy) and expectations (lose 4 lbs in 4 weeks) • makes assumptions about her exercise or diet

B. Clinical management skills	Positive indicators:
• Recognition and management of common medical conditions in primary care. Demonstrates flexible and structured approach to decision making • Demonstrating ability to deal with multiple complaints and co-morbidity and to promote a shared approach to managing problems Maps on the blueprint to: • **Management (B)** • **Co-morbidity and health promotion (C)**	• clarifies for patient that 'herbal' is not synonymous with 'safe' • discusses options for weight loss and sets realistic goals • encourages and supports healthy and sustainable lifestyle changes • promotes a therapeutic relationship and safety-nets Negative indicators: • fails to address safety and efficacy issues • is prescriptive or sets unrealistic goals • prescribes or refers inappropriately • fails to promote the doctor–patient relationship and discourages further consultations
C. Interpersonal skills	Positive indicators:
• Use of recognised communication techniques that enhance understanding of a patient's illness and promote a shared approach to managing problems • Practising ethically with respect for equality and diversity in line with accepted codes of professional conduct Maps on the blueprint to: • **Person-centred approach (D)** • **Professional attitude (E)**	• is sensitive but thorough in exploring the patient's ideas, concerns and expectations • understands the whole person not just her social anxiety • forms a shared understanding with the patient regarding her perception of herself • provides ongoing health promotion – encourages a healthy lifestyle • promotes a therapeutic relationship – is welcoming, facilitative and empowering Negative indicators: • is insensitive, rude or patronising • runs through the 'obesity management' protocol • does not achieve 'shared understanding' – there is a discrepancy between doctor and patient agendas • promotes 'quick fix' measures • promotes excessive reliance on the doctor or inappropriately discourages further consultations

Debrief

- What could you learn from this consultation? How to:
  - establish rapport, by showing a genuine interest in the patient's life within 30 seconds of meeting
  - invite the patient to tell her story – being facilitative and open
  - acknowledge the reason for her attendance, so that she knows you know why she is attending
  - identify her specific concerns and clarify her expectations
  - wind down the discussion, with sentences such as *"how do you feel about it now?"*
- What questions would you ask to 'understand the whole person, not the disease'?
- How would you phrase your health promotion advice?
- How would you develop a therapeutic doctor–patient relationship?

Relevant literature

For information on internet printouts, see:
www.jmir.org/2002/1/e5/

Brown H (2003) Patient with bundle of printouts from the internet. *Pulse*, 24 Nov:
www.pulsetoday.co.uk and search for 'bundle of printouts'.

Little P, Everitt H, Williamson I, *et al.* (2001) Preferences of patients for patient centred approach to consultation in primary care: observational study. *BMJ*, **322**: 468–472:
www.bmj.com/cgi/reprint/322/7284/468

Potts HW, Wyatt JC (2002) Survey of doctors' experience of patients using the internet. *J Med Internet Res*, **4**(1): e5.
www.bmj.com/cgi/reprint/321/7254/165

Video 10 – Hypnotherapy

Brief to the doctor

Mrs KJ is a 41 year old woman who requests hypnotherapy. She used to see Dr Brown, now retired, for hypnotherapy.

Patient summary

Name   KJ

Date of birth (Age)   41

Past medical history   Contraception (4 months ago)
                            Acute on chronic low back pain (6 months ago)
                            CT head – no acute changes (14 months ago)
                            Severe head injury with frontal lobe damage (18 years ago)

Repeat medication   Microgynon once daily × 126T (4 months ago)

Tasks for the doctor

This case is written to test how the candidate deals with a request for treatment that is not available on the NHS. The case is weighted to assess the doctor's interpersonal skills, that is, his ability to 'give bad news' and deal with the patient's emotions.

Although the framework for 'breaking bad news' has historically been used in consultations communicating the poor prognosis of an illness, the framework can be adapted to consultations in which the patient is given news they do not want to hear, such as the unavailability of certain treatments on the NHS.

Read the guidance on how to communicate bad news and a brief overview of hypnotherapy. Then watch the DVD and mark the case.

For information on how to break bad news, see Faulkner (1998).
- Give bad news in a sensitive manner and at the individual's pace.
- Allow some time before attempting to explore feelings and identify concerns.
- Discuss issues honestly. This may reassure the patient; help him to plan; readjust his hopes and aims.
- Check the reason for the requests directed to you, for example, *"Why the request for hypnotherapy?"*
- Show interest in patient's ideas, for example, *"I wonder if you'd considered any other treatments?"*

- Confirm or elaborate – for example, *"what do you mean by 'a wreck'?"*
- Acknowledge and legitimise the emotion, show concern and remain calm. Displays of emotion from the patient should not be seen as a personal attack.

For information on hypnotherapy, see www.mercurysky.co.uk/bsmdh/faq.htm.

- In therapy, the client relaxes deeply, his attention narrows down, and he focuses on suggestions made by the therapist.
- The suggestions may be aimed at helping the person change the way he responds to a situation, for example, he may be asked to visualise himself taking deep breaths and feeling calm in a confined space.
- Self-hypnotic suggestions may help control anxiety and stress by building self-confidence.
- If a patient lives within the catchment area of a NHS doctor who uses hypnosis, then treatment on the NHS is possible.

Having read the above guidance, watch case 10 on the DVD. Mark the candidate according to the schedule listed below.

Generic indicators for targeted assessment domains	Descriptors – positive and negative
A. Data gathering, technical and assessment skills • Gathering of data for clinical judgement, choice of examination, investigations and their interpretations • Demonstrating proficiency in performing physical examinations and using diagnostic and therapeutic instruments Maps on the blueprint to: • **Data gathering and interpretation (A)** • **Technical skills (F)**	Positive indicators: • explores the reasons for the patient's request • elicits the patient's ideas (she prefers hypnotherapy to anxiolytics for CT scans), concerns (who is going to do the hypnotherapy) and expectations (help in finding a hypnotherapist) • finds out how the problem affects the patient socially – effect on work and relationships • explores the patient's willingness to try alternative therapies Negative indicators: • does not allow the patient to express their fears about having a CT scan • does not identify the patient's health beliefs • does not identify the psycho-social impact of the patient's anxiety • does not explore options in a way that moves the consultation forward, for example, says *"I'll check and get back to you"*

B. Clinical management skills • Recognition and management of common medical conditions in primary care. Demonstrates flexible and structured approach to decision making. • Demonstrating ability to deal with multiple complaints and co-morbidity and to promote a shared approach to managing problems Maps on the blueprint to: • **Management (B)** • **Co-morbidity and health promotion (C)**	Positive indicators: • clarifies for patient that he cannot arrange NHS hypnotherapy • helps the patient plan • shows interest in the patient's ideas, thereby empowering the patient and promoting a therapeutic relationship Negative indicators: • fails to tackle the issue or delays giving the 'bad' news • does not explore solutions to the problem • dismisses the patient's ideas and/or prescribes or refers inappropriately • fails to build a cordial and therapeutic doctor–patient relationship
C. Interpersonal skills • Use of recognised communication techniques that enhances understanding of a patient's illness and promotes a shared approach to managing problems • Practising ethically with respect for equality and diversity in line with accepted codes of professional conduct Maps on the blueprint to: • **Person-centred approach (D)** • **Professional attitude (E)**	Positive indicators: • appears sensitive and is led by the patient, that is, information is dripped according to the patient's readiness • seems honest and empathetic • shows genuine concern for the patient's well-being • behaves professionally • appears facilitative, empowering and supportive Negative indicators: • appears blunt, callous or put-upon • appears dishonest or tactless • acts in an uncaring or unconcerned manner • displays impatience, awkwardness or anger • seems dismissive or unwelcoming

Debrief

- What could you learn from this consultation? How to:
  - 'drip' information at the patient's pace
  - facilitate an expression of emotion – use open questions and reflective statements
  - listen actively and respond warmly, demonstrating concern for the patient
  - be professional, courteous and calm when confronted with the patient's emotion
  - be honest about the lack of resources
  - provide on-going support and follow-up, if required
- How would you assess the patient's pace?
- What questions would you ask to uncover the patient's emotions?
- How would you say no, for example, when asked for aesthetic plastic surgery or osteopathy on the NHS?
- How would you demonstrate support to the patient having just informed them that they could not have a particular treatment?

Relevant literature

Faulkner A (1998) ABC of palliative care: Communication with patients, families, and other professionals, *BMJ*; **316**: 130–132, see: www.bmj.com/cgi/content/full/316/7125/130.

For a case study on hypnotherapy for anxiety, see: www.hypnos.co.uk/hypnomag/howard2.htm.

Video 11 - Diarrhoea

Brief to the doctor

Miss TD is a 20 year old woman who presents with diarrhoea.

Patient summary

Name	TD
Date of birth (Age)	20
Past medical history	Chest infection (1 week ago) Contraception (3 months ago)
Medication	Amoxicillin 250 mg thrice daily × 15T Yasmin once daily × 126T (3 months ago)

Tasks for the doctor

This case is written to test how the candidate deals with a common presentation in general practice. The case assesses the doctor's ability to deal with the clinical problem (diarrhoea) and the subsidiary concerns, namely, occupational and family planning issues.

Read the guidance on how to assess antibiotic-associated diarrhoea, manage gastroenteritis and advise on contraception. Then watch the DVD and mark the case.

For information on how to assess antibiotic-associated diarrhoea, see:
www.emedicine.com/MED/topic3412.htm
- *Clostridium difficile* (CD) produces spores which, when ingested into a human gut, develop into mature bacteria. Antibiotics, by killing off gut commensals, allow the number of CD to increase and this causes problems. CD produce toxins, which cause inflammation, mainly to the large bowel.
- Most cases occur in hospitalised patients.
- Symptoms include mild or moderate watery diarrhoea, crampy abdominal pain, nausea and fever.
- Symptoms start within a few days of starting the antibiotic. However, in some cases symptoms develop up to 10 weeks after finishing a course of antibiotics.
- In mild or moderate diarrhoea, stopping the antibiotic may be the only treatment needed.

For information on managing gastroenteritis, see www.cks.library.nhs.uk/gastroenteritis.

- Red flags in a healthy adult are diarrhoea lasting for more than a fortnight, bloody diarrhoea, pyrexia or recent foreign travel.
- Examine for dehydration, appendicitis and acute abdomen.
- Food handlers, who handle unwrapped or raw food, must be clear of symptoms for at least 48 hours before returning to work.

For information on contraception, see the Faculty of Family Planning guidance. The general advice for women using combined oral contraception who have persistent vomiting or severe diarrhoea for more than 24 hours is to follow the instructions for missed pills (see the 'missed pills' flowchart on pages 10 and 11 of: www.fsrh.org/pdfs/archive/FirstPrescCombOralCont06.pdf and also www.fsrh.org/pdfs/CEUStatementMissedPills.pdf).

Having read the above guidance, watch case 11 on the DVD. Mark the candidate according to the schedule listed below.

Generic indicators for targeted assessment domains	Descriptors – positive and negative
A. Data gathering, technical and assessment skills - Gathering of data for clinical judgement, choice of examination, investigations and their interpretations - Demonstrating proficiency in performing physical examinations and using diagnostic and therapeutic instruments Maps on the blueprint to: - **Data gathering and interpretation (A)** - **Technical skills (F)**	Positive indicators: - explores the patient's health beliefs, that is, what the patient thinks is causing the diarrhoea - excludes 'red flags' - elicits the patient's concerns (regarding her fitness to handle food and be well for her holiday) - performs a targeted abdominal examination and correctly interprets findings Negative indicators: - does not explore the patient's belief that her antibiotics have caused the diarrhoea - does not exclude red flags - does not elicit the patient's concerns - does not perform a targeted examination and/or is incorrect in interpretation of the findings

B. Clinical management skills • Recognition and management of common medical conditions in primary care. Demonstrates flexible and structured approach to decision making. • Demonstrating ability to deal with multiple complaints and co-morbidity and to promote a shared approach to managing problems Maps on the blueprint to: • **Management (B)** • **Co-morbidity and health promotion (C)**	Positive indicators: • explains the diagnosis in appropriate language • the explanation incorporates the patient's health beliefs • involves the patient in the management plan • management is evidence-based Negative indicators: • fails to explain the diagnosis or uses jargon the patient is unlikely to understand • the patient's health beliefs are not addressed • the patient is not given an opportunity to be involved in the management plan • management is not appropriate for the working diagnosis or not in line with current accepted UK general practice
C. Interpersonal skills • Use of recognised communication techniques that enhances understanding of a patient's illness and promotes a shared approach to managing problems • Practising ethically with respect for equality and diversity in line with accepted codes of professional conduct Maps on the blueprint to: • **Person-centred approach (D)** • **Professional attitude (E)**	Positive indicators: • appears empathetic to the patient's condition • shows interest in understanding the patient's concerns – is holistic • if medication is prescribed, the patient is correctly advised on how to take the medication • ascertains whether the patient's concerns and queries were addressed Negative indicators: • appears insensitive or uncaring about the patient's condition • appears uninterested in or dismissive of the patient's agenda • if medication is prescribed, the patient is not advised or is incorrectly advised on how to take the medication • fails to confirm mutual agreement

Debrief

- What could you learn from this consultation? How to:
  - explore the patient's ideas, concerns and expectations
  - systematically explore 'red flags'
  - target the examination and relay findings in appropriate language
  - construct a management plan in line with current accepted UK practice
  - appropriately address occupational issues
  - make effective use of resources (time and investigations)
- What would you examine for? Are you able to perform the examination slickly?
- How would you address the patient's health beliefs in your explanation?
- How would you deal with the patient's request for antibiotics, or a sick note?
- How would you encourage concordance?

Relevant literature

For information on gastroenteritis, see:
www.cks.library.nhs.uk/gastroenteritis.

For information on antibiotic-associated diarrhoea (*Clostridium difficile*), see:
www.emedicine.com/MED/topic3412.htm.

For guidance on management of infections in primary care, see:
www.hpa.org.uk/webc/HPAwebFile/HPAweb_C/1194947333801.

For an excellent website detailing the examination of the abdomen, see:
http://meded.ucsd.edu/clinicalmed/abdomen.htm#Topical.

Video 12 – Febrile convulsion

Brief to the doctor

Mrs BC is a 35 year old woman who presents for information about her daughter Millie's condition. Millie is 9 months old.

Patient summary

Name	Millie C
Date of birth (Age)	9 months
Past medical history	Up to date with childhood immunisations
	Normal development to date
Repeat medication	None recorded

Tasks for the doctor

This case is written to test how the candidate deals with an anxious mum who is seeking reassurance and further information about her daughter's prognosis. The case assesses the doctor's ability to discuss risk or likelihood of recurrence and allay maternal anxiety.

Read the guidance on how to assess childhood seizures and reassure effectively. Then watch the DVD and mark the case.

For information on febrile seizures, see Offringa and Moyer (2001).
- A febrile convulsion is a seizure occurring in a child aged 6 months to 5 years, associated with fever arising from infection or inflammation outside the central nervous system in a child who is otherwise neurologically normal.
- 90% occur between 6 months and 3 years.
- The four most common causes are viral infections, otitis media, tonsillitis, and urinary tract infections.
- Current UK practice for the management of febrile seizures include paracetamol, ibuprofen, tepid sponging. Advise parents not to force anything into the mouth when the child is fitting.
- Refer children under 18 months, those with features of meningitis, multiple fits, prolonged fits lasting longer than 15 minutes, systemically unwell children and where parents are anxious or unable to cope.
- Only 1% of children who have had a febrile convulsion go on to develop epilepsy compared with 0.4% who have not.
- The risk of recurrence with simple febrile seizures is 10%.

For information on reassuring patients, see Donovan and Blake (2000).

- Reassurance is an important part of consultations, whether the diagnosis is clear or uncertain.
- Clinicians assume that patients are reassured by clear and confident statements about the diagnosis or the failure to find disease, with patients who remain anxious after such reassurance at risk of being labelled as neurotic or having abnormal illness behaviour.
- Clinicians try, ineffectively, to reduce anxiety by emphasising the mildness, early stage, or non-seriousness of the disorder and the likelihood that patients would recover.
- Effective reassurance acknowledges the patients' problems and incorporates their health beliefs. For examples of explanations patients found reassuring, consult the original article.

Having read the above guidance, watch case 12 on the DVD. Mark the candidate according to the schedule listed below.

Generic indicators for targeted assessment domains	Descriptors – positive and negative
A. Data gathering, technical and assessment skills • Gathering of data for clinical judgement, choice of examination, investigations and their interpretations • Demonstrating proficiency in performing physical examinations and using diagnostic and therapeutic instruments Maps on the blueprint to: • **Data gathering and interpretation (A)** • **Technical skills (F)**	Positive indicators: • encourages mum to provide an account of what happened • obtains sufficient information about the seizure and hospital treatment to exclude need for review, re-examination or referral of Millie • obtains the relevant social information to place the complaint in context Negative indicators: • does not encourage the mum to tell her story – is dismissive, interrupts, or discourages the flow of the story • does not obtain information to exclude need for review, re-examination or referral of Millie – assumes that Millie has been treated appropriately and is fine • does not obtain the relevant social information to place the complaint in context – does not obtain the information about mum's brother

B. Clinical management skills • Recognition and management of common medical conditions in primary care. Demonstrates flexible and structured approach to decision making. • Demonstrating ability to deal with multiple complaints and co-morbidity and to promote a shared approach to managing problems Maps on the blueprint to: • **Management (B)** • **Co-morbidity and health promotion (C)**	Positive indicators: • explains the diagnosis in appropriate language – clarifies what a febrile seizure is • the explanation builds on the patient's health belief that different illness can cause fever • involves mum in the management plan – mum is given a clear outline of what to do in future febrile illnesses • management is evidence-based – appropriate antipyretics are advised Negative indicators: • fails to explain the diagnosis or uses jargon mum is unlikely to understand • the explanation does not incorporate mum's health belief • mum is not given an opportunity to be involved in the management plan – mum is simply advised to consult again if Millie is ill without any advice on practical measures she could take before consulting • management is not appropriate for the working diagnosis or not in line with current accepted UK general practice
C. Interpersonal skills • Use of recognised communication techniques that enhances understanding of a patient's illness and promotes a shared approach to managing problems • Practising ethically with respect for equality and diversity in line with accepted codes of professional conduct Maps on the blueprint to: • **Person-centred approach (D)** • **Professional attitude (E)**	Positive indicators: • identified and addressed the mum's concerns about risk of recurrence and risk of epilepsy • identified and addressed the mum's expectation for advice on what to do if a 2nd seizure occurs • appears empathetic and interested; is reassuring • ascertains whether mum's concerns and queries were addressed Negative indicators: • does not identify and/or does not address the mum's concerns about risk of recurrence and risk of epilepsy – is dismissive of concerns or implies that the hospital should have provided this information • does not identify and/or does not address the mum's expectation for advice on what to do if a 2nd seizure occurs • appears dismissive or uninterested; does not reassure mum or increase her confidence • terminates the consultation without confirming satisfaction with the discussion or understanding of the information given

Debrief

- What could you learn from this consultation? How to:
  - encourage the patient, verbally and non-verbally, to tell the story
  - negotiate the agenda: *"there are two issues here: firstly, what happened last night and secondly, your concerns about recurrence"*
  - screen for information to exclude the need for review, re-examination or referral
  - assess the patient's starting point – *"You are an experienced mum. How would you..."*
  - acknowledge the patient's feelings and reassure effectively
  - elicit mum's reactions and feelings to the information given
  - check with the mum to see that plans have been accepted and concerns addressed
  - make effective use of resources (time and investigations)
- Review the DVD, particularly mum's description of the seizure, to identify statements that are unclear. How would you clarify these statements?
- How could you periodically summarise to verify your understanding of what mum has said?
- How would you express concern, understanding and a willingness to help?
- How would you encourage mum's contribution to the management plan?
- How would you close the session?

Relevant literature

For information on febrile seizures, see:
Offringa M and Moyer VA (2001) Evidence based paediatrics: Evidence based management of seizures associated with fever. *BMJ*, **323**: 1111–1114:
www.bmj.com/cgi/content/full/323/7321/1111

http://cks.library.nhs.uk/febrile_seizure/management/detailed_answers/assessing_a_child_who_has_had_a_febrile_seizure#

For information on medical reassurance, see:
Donovan JL and Blake RB (2000) Qualitative study of interpretation of reassurance among patients attending rheumatology clinics: *"just a touch of arthritis, doctor?"*
BMJ, **320**: 541–544:
www.bmj.com/cgi/content/full/320/7234/541

Edwards A, Elwyn G, and Mulley A (2002) Explaining risks: turning numerical data into meaningful pictures, *BMJ*, **324**: 827–830:
www.bmj.com/content/324/7341/827.1.full

Video 13 – Allergy test

Brief to the doctor

Mr JH is a 23 year old man who requests allergy testing.

Patient summary

Name	JH
Date of birth (Age)	23
Past medical history	Sprained ankle (L) 8 months ago Sprained wrist (R) 3 years ago
Repeat medication	None

Tasks for the doctor

This case is written to test how the candidate deals with a request for treatment that is available on the NHS but may not be clinically indicated for the patient requesting the test. The case is weighted to assess the doctor's interpersonal skills, that is, his ability to analyse need, negotiate with patients and make effective use of resources. Patients often request tests because of perceived needs. Good communicators are able to elicit the reasons for requests and deal with these (usually emotional) issues tactfully.

Read the guidance on how to make effective use of resources and communicate well with emotional issues. Then watch the DVD and mark the case.

For information on how to make effective use of resources, see *Commissioning Report* (Nov 07):

Key issues that need consideration by clinicians when making requests for individual treatments or procedures:
- that a significant clinical need has been identified
- effective benefit has been established
- alternative treatments have been considered
- the safety and efficacy of the product
- proven clinical evidence
- exceptional circumstances
- cost that may be incurred
- risks have been identified

- the issue of informed consent has been addressed
- National Institute for Health and Clinical Excellence (NICE) guidance
- local guidance
- in addition to the above, consideration should be given to the likelihood of measurable improvement in the quality of life of the individuals that would be receiving the treatments or procedures
- requests for funding may also be made for treatments or procedures in relation to individual exceptional circumstances on the grounds that their condition is causing psychological ill health and social isolation

Making effective use of resources (RCGP):

The excellent GP	**The unacceptable GP**
• Only prescribes treatments which make an effective contribution to the patient's overall management • Takes resources into account when choosing between treatments of similar effectiveness	• Consistently prescribes unnecessary or ineffective treatments • Takes no note of resources when choosing between similar treatments • Refuses to register patients whose treatment may be costly

For information on how to communicate effectively with emotional issues, see Buckman (2002).

The central technique of acknowledging and addressing emotions is straightforward. The empathic response, for example, is a technique that consists of three steps:

1. identifying the emotion
2. identifying the source of the emotion
3. responding in a way that shows you have made the connection between the first two steps

Having read the above guidance, watch case 13 on the DVD. Mark the candidate according to the schedule listed below.

Generic indicators for targeted assessment domains	Descriptors – positive and negative
A. Data gathering, technical and assessment skills • Gathering of data for clinical judgement, choice of examination, investigations and their interpretations • Demonstrating proficiency in performing physical examinations and using diagnostic and therapeutic instruments Maps on the blueprint to: • **Data gathering and interpretation (A)** • **Technical skills (F)**	Positive indicators: • explores the reasons for the patient's request • elicits the patient's ideas (his symptoms are caused by allergies), concerns (his wife wants pets or a baby) and expectations (an NHS allergy test) • finds out how the problem affects the patient socially – effect on work and relationships • obtains sufficient information to exclude a significant allergic reaction or medical problem Negative indicators: • fails to elicit important parts of the history, such as the reason for the request • does not identify the patient's health beliefs • does not place the request in a psychological or social context • does not obtain sufficient information to exclude a significant allergic reaction or medical problem – makes assumptions • undertakes inappropriate or inadequate examinations
B. Clinical management skills • Recognition and management of common medical conditions in primary care. Demonstrates flexible and structured approach to decision making. • Demonstrating ability to deal with multiple complaints and co-morbidity and to promote a shared approach to managing problems Maps on the blueprint to: • **Management (B)** • **Co-morbidity and health promotion (C)**	Positive indicators: • gives information about allergic reactions and testing in assimilable chunks • clarifies for patient that the request for testing depends on clinical need and intended benefit • takes into account 'exceptional' circumstances Negative indicators: • fails to be guided by the patient's response when giving information about allergic reactions and testing • does not explain why the test is not being arranged • undertakes inappropriate investigations • gives treatments that are inconsistent with best practice or evidence

C. Interpersonal skills	Positive indicators:
• Use of recognised communication techniques that enhances understanding of a patient's illness and promotes a shared approach to managing problems • Practising ethically with respect for equality and diversity in line with accepted codes of professional conduct Maps on the blueprint to: • **Person-centred approach (D)** • **Professional attitude (E)**	• demonstrates active listening and appears sensitive • explores important issues using open and closed questioning • seems understanding • encourages the patient's contribution: the patient feels comfortable to ask questions, seek clarification or express doubts • checks with the patient that plans are accepted and concerns addressed Negative indicators: • consistently ignores, interrupts, or contradicts the patient; appears insensitive • is unable to facilitate the patient's response and clarify issues such that important issues are missed • seems unable to discuss sensitive or personal matters; may act uncaring or unconcerned • displays impatience, awkwardness or anger – the patient feels unable to ask questions, seek clarification or express doubts • does not negotiate with the patient or the patient is given little opportunity to be involved in the management plan

Debrief

- What could you learn from this consultation? How to:
  - take time to listen to patients, and allow them to express their own concerns
  - consider relevant psychological and social factors as well as physical ones
  - use clear language appropriate for the patient
  - use investigations when they will help management of the condition – assess clinical need, intended benefit and exceptional circumstances
  - make sound management decisions which are based on good practice and evidence
- How would you facilitate the expression of a patient's concerns or emotions?
- What questions would you ask to uncover the patient's social circumstances or concerns?
- How would you explain to a patient that an MRI scan for mechanical back pain is not currently needed?
- How would you explore the 'exceptional circumstances' in a patient requesting NHS plastic surgery, such as laser treatment for a facial haemangioma?

Relevant literature

For an example of 'An effective use of resources report', see:
Commissioning Report (Nov 07) by Bury NHS PCT: www.medlaw.eu/pdf/Bury.PCT.
IFR.29.11.10.pdf

See: www.rcgp-curriculum.org.uk/curriculum_documents/gp_curriculum_
statements.aspx especially www.rcgp-curriculum.org.uk/pdf/curr_3_3_Clinical_
ethics.pdf

For information on communicating with emotional issues, see:
Buckman R (2002) Communications and emotions, *BMJ*; **325**: 672:
www.bmj.com/cgi/content/full/325/7366/672

Learning consultation skills for COT and CSA

The aim of this section of the book is to encourage readers to practise patient consultations in preparation for COT and CSA. The reader is required to work out the necessary questions and conduct a 'consultation'.

Each of the 20 cases comprises the following sections.
- *'Summary of the patient'*, including any recent test results – the basic background you need.
- *'Tasks for the doctor'* – what you are expected to establish in the consultation.
- *'More about the patient'* – more about the patient's background and presentation; this section can be used by a study partner to allow them to act as the 'patient'.
- *'Approach to be taken'* – this explains what the examiners are assessing with the case and provides a model answer.
- *'Test your theoretical knowledge'* – a short series of single answer multiple choice questions to test how well you understand current clinical practice; answers are provided at the end of the book.
- Each case ends with suggestions for further reading.

There are two ways to use this section of the book.
1. Ideally, you will work through the cases with a study partner, with one of you assuming the role of 'patient' and the other the role of 'doctor'.
    - The 'patient' reads the first two pages of the case, comprising the *Summary of the patient* and *More about the patient* sections – this allows them to understand the expectations of the patient so they can then answer the doctor's questions.
    - The 'doctor' should read only the first page comprising the *Summary of the patient* and should then conduct a consultation with the patient with a view to:
    A. gathering data to get to the nub of the problem
    B. managing the clinical problem
    C. demonstrating their interpersonal skills

2. Working alone, read through the first page and then note down the questions you would wish to ask in the consultation, referring to the *More about the patient* section as necessary. You may wish to use a COT *pro forma* for your answers.

COT *pro forma*[1]

A. Data gathering, examination and clinical assessment skills

1. **Define the clinical problem:**
   - What questions do you ask to clarify why the patient has presented today?
   - How would you explore the patient's ideas, concerns, expectations and health beliefs?

2. **Perform an appropriate physical or mental examination**
   - What is the appropriate targeted physical or mental state examination?
   - Can you perform the examination slickly and sensitively using appropriate medical equipment?

B. Clinical management skills

3. **Make an appropriate working diagnosis**
   - On the basis of probability, what is your working diagnosis?

4. **Explain the problem to the patient using appropriate language**
   - How would you explain the diagnosis to the patient?
   - Is your explanation jargon-free, well organised and logical?
   - Does it address the patient's concerns and expectations?

5. **Provide holistic care and use resources effectively**
   - Was your management plan informed by national or local guidelines?
   - Have you referred appropriately?

6. **Prescribe appropriately**
   - Have you considered drug interactions or discussed side effects?
   - Did you check the patient's understanding of the medication?

7. **Specify the conditions and interval for follow-up**
   - Have you safety netted appropriately?

---

1   Adapted from a COT *pro forma* developed by Dr David Chadwick, Springfield Surgery, Oxfordshire.

C. Interpersonal skills: know and treat this patient

8. Achieve rapport
- Have you demonstrated active listening, sensitivity, and empathy?
- Have you used the patient's ideas and beliefs in explanations?
- Have you addressed the patient's specific concerns and expectations?

9. Give the patient the opportunity to be involved in significant management decisions
- Have you involved the patient in decisions?
- Have you negotiated, offered various treatment options or encouraged autonomy and opinions?

Case 1 – Menopausal symptoms

Brief to the doctor

Mrs JS is a 51 year old woman who presents for treatment of her hot flushes. She used HRT tablets 2 years ago for peri-menopausal flushing and stopped 3 months ago after developing PV bleeding. Her hysteroscopy 1 month ago was negative. Having discontinued with the HRT 3 months ago, the flushes have recurred.

Patient summary

Name	JS
Date of birth (Age)	51
Social and Family History	Married, two children
Past medical history	Hysteroscopy (1 month ago) – no pathology
	Postmenopausal bleeding on HRT (3 months ago)
	Hip pain (1 year ago)
	Menopausal symptoms (flushing) for 2 years
Current medication	Ibuprofen 400 mg prn × 84

Blood tests   Tests were done 1 month ago (pre-hysteroscopy)

Plasma fasting glucose	5 mmol/l (3.65–5.5)
Fasting cholesterol	5 mmol/l
TSH	1.12
Hb	13.2 g/dl (13–17)
MCV	86 (83–105)
BMI	25.6
BP	117/60

Tasks for the doctor

In this case, the tasks are to:
- present Mrs JS with suitable treatment options for her hot flushes
- provide her with sufficient information to make an informed decision
- prescribe appropriately

Brief to the patient – more about the patient

1. Profile:

- Mrs JS a 51 year old woman
- married with 2 children, ages 18 and 15
- a paediatric out-patient nurse
- flushing is becoming a real nuisance: disturbs sleep, embarrasses her when it occurs at work and she feels tired
- she felt well on HRT but really disliked having a hysteroscopy for PMB so, if possible, would prefer not to restart HRT; she's read about soya and yams but is unaware of other treatment options

2. She is seeing the doctor today because:

- she has not had a period or any PV bleeding for 3 months; prior to this, she had withdrawal bleeds on the HRT
- she is not keen on hormone treatments or the Mirena coil; she does not have any other health problems and uses condoms for contraception
- she is now flushing more than three times per day every other day – her sleep is interrupted and she feels tired
- she is worried about her ability to maintain a calm and reassuring demeanour at work (paediatric OPD) if she continues to feel tired and irritable
- she expects the doctor to give her advice about complementary therapies, prescribe something or refer her to the Menopause Clinic – she wants an action plan for this problem and is not happy with a 'wait and see' policy
- she quickly grasps the medical information imparted and nods her head to indicate understanding of the treatment options
- if she feels coerced into choosing one option (such as HRT), she asks for a referral to the Menopause Clinic
- if the doctor laughs at her health beliefs, she challenges him on his views on complementary therapies
- if the doctor offers her SSRIs, at first she seems sceptical and asks if the doctor thinks she is depressed – she accepts this treatment after a discussion on its evidence, efficacy and safety

Approach to be taken

A. Data gathering, examination and clinical assessment skills

1. *Define the clinical problem: clarify why the patient has presented today*
   The doctor:
   - reads the patient summary provided prior to seeing Mrs JS
   - detects Mrs JS's reluctance to restart HRT and her eagerness to explore alternative treatment options for her menopausal flushing
   - asks open questions to explore the frequency, severity, impact of the flushing, and her specific concerns about HRT
   - asks closed questions to ascertain the presence (or absence) of other menopausal symptoms, including periods
   - excludes red flags, such as on-going PMB
   - elicits how the problem affects Mrs JS at work (and at home)
   - discovers Mrs JS's ideas regarding phytoestrogens
   - discovers her concerns about further episodes of PMB on HRT
   - discovers her expectations for further treatment, either conventional or complementary
   - summarises the problem: *"Mrs JS, on stopping your HRT you have experienced flushes that interfere with your ability to work comfortably. You'd prefer not to take HRT and would like me to discuss alternative treatment options with you. Have I understood you correctly?"*

2. *Perform an appropriate physical or mental examination*
   - In this case, neither a formal physical or mental state examination is required.

B. Clinical management skills

3. *Make an appropriate working diagnosis*
   The doctor, based on the history and exclusion of 'red flags', makes a clinically sound working diagnosis – menopausal flushing.

4. *Explain the problem to the patient using appropriate language*
   The doctor:
   - explains that the menopausal flushing is a 'nuisance' problem rather than a 'serious health problem'
   - agrees with Mrs JS that it should be treated to improve her quality of life
   - discusses in jargon-free language the benefits and risks of HRT (IUS + oestrogen only HRT), SSRIs, and phytoestrogens; may briefly mention 2nd and 3rd line alternatives such venlafaxine, gabapentin or clonidine which can be initiated if recommended by the Menopause Clinic
   - provides information in adequate chunks and checks understanding at each step

- uses the patient's ideas: phytoestrogens may be useful; however, there is little clinical evidence regarding their efficacy and safety (see www.rcn.org.uk/__data/assets/pdf_file/0007/78712/003069.pdf)
- addresses the patient's concerns: further PMB on HRT may require investigation to exclude endometrial pathology, hence endometrial protection with an IUS and oestrogen-only HRT or SSRIs may be more acceptable to the patient
- addresses the patient's expectations – provides treatment options

5. *Provide holistic care and use resources effectively*
The doctor:
- may use or discuss complementary medicines, such as Red Clover and Black Cohosh
- may use time as a therapeutic tool: if Mrs JS seems to have difficulty in making a decision regarding which treatment she would prefer, the doctor could offer a leaflet and provide a follow-up appointment
- offers the treatment options and, if Mrs JS indicates that she would like to get her treatment sorted out today, helps her to choose the most appropriate therapy for her
- demonstrates practice of evidence-based medicine – he discusses which treatment options have a good evidence base and are proven to be effective
- is informed by national or local guidelines – www.cks.library.nhs.uk/ menopause

6. *Prescribe appropriately*
The doctor:
- if prescribing SSRIs, chooses a cost-effective medication
- prescribes the appropriate dose and number of tablets
- discusses drug interactions and side effects
- checks the patient's understanding of the medication

7. *Specify the conditions and interval for follow-up*
The doctor:
- safety-nets appropriately – when to consult again and why: *"Is it OK to meet again in a fortnight to check how you are getting on with this tablet? Obviously, if there are problems, I'd like to see you sooner."*

C. Interpersonal skills: know and treat this patient

8. *Achieve rapport*
The doctor:
- listens attentively to the patient's request for treatment and her concerns regarding PMB on HRT
- displays empathy to the adverse effect flushing has on her confidence and comfort at work

- is non-judgemental about the patient's health beliefs regarding complementary therapies
- addresses the patient's specific concerns and expectations, for example, does not spend more time speaking about HRT and breast cancer when this is not the patient's specific concern; addresses her concern about the difficulty in differentiating between significant endometrial pathology and 'nuisance' break-through bleeding on HRT

9. *Give the patient the opportunity to be involved in significant management decisions*
The doctor:
- shares a raft of management options and involves the patient in decisions
- negotiates with the patient which option may be better for her given her specific concern (HRT and BTB)
- reassures the patient SSRIs are effective in reducing the frequency of flushing and are not, in this instance, being used to treat a psychological problem
- encourages autonomy and opinions – with regard to complementary therapies, the doctor provides a balanced discussion regarding evidence, cost, etc., but refrains from making derogatory comments if he does not share these health beliefs

Debrief

Discuss how the doctor could, if needed, improve his performance. In particular, assess whether the doctor:

- empathised? If so, how?
- presented the patient with appropriate treatment options?
- explained the risks and benefits of treatments in simple language?

If the consultation over-ran:

- how could the history taking be shortened?
- how could the explanations be simplified?
- how could the doctor have expressed empathy and understanding? Comment on the doctor's non-verbal behaviour and his summarising.

Revising data gathering

Are there any existing medical records for the doctor to peruse before the patient consults?

- The doctor was given a patient summary prior to the patient's presentation.

What questions could the doctor ask to discover the patient's ideas, concerns, expectations and health beliefs?

- Ideas: *"I understand that you are not keen to restart HRT. Were there any other treatments you had in mind?"*
- Concerns: *"You don't seem keen on using SSRIs. Are there particular concerns you have about these tablets?"*
- Expectations: *"It seems to me the flushing is really interfering with your work and you want to discuss the risks and benefits of potential treatments. Shall we run through these options?"*
- Health beliefs: *"You know that SSRIs are used to treat depression. What you may not know is that they are also particularly useful in reducing the frequency of menopausal flushing; it is not being used as an antidepressant here. In addition, there is no added risk of BTB with SSRIs, unlike HRT."*

Once the doctor has gathered sufficient information, how could he summarise the problem for the patient?

- *"Mrs JS, you have given me quite a lot of information. I'd like to summarise our discussion back to you so you can correct me if I've left out anything important."*
- *"You suffer from menopausal flushing. You have used HRT in the past but unfortunately developed BTB. You would like treatment of the flushing, but you would prefer to consider options other than HRT. In particular, you'd like to discuss the effectiveness and safety of natural oestrogens."*

Test your theoretical knowledge

For each of the following statements, answer true (T) or false (F).

1. For vasomotor symptoms, consider a 2 week trial of paroxetine (40 mg daily).
2. For vasomotor symptoms, consider a 2 week trial of citalopram (20 mg daily).
3. Venlafaxine 37.5 mg twice a day is licensed for the treatment of menopausal flushing.
4. There is evidence that smoking cigarettes increases the likelihood of flushing.
5. Ginseng, black cohosh, and red clover may be used in women with contraindications to oestrogen (e.g. breast cancer).

Relevant literature

http://cks.library.nhs.uk/menopause/in_depth/management_issues

Case 2 - Neck pain

Brief to the doctor

Mr AB is a 34 year old man who presents to your surgery with a 4 week history of neck pain that is getting progressively worse.

Patient summary

Name	AB
Date of birth (Age)	34
Social and family history	Single Lives with mother
Past medical history	Road traffic accident 17 years ago • Fracture of right femur and tibial plateau • Fracture of left ankle
Current medication	None

Investigations   2 years ago:
   BMI   34
   BP   135/90
   Urine   NAD on Multistix

Tasks for the doctor

In this case, the tasks are to:
- clarify the neck pain symptoms, identify causative factors (occupational history), perform an appropriate examination, formulate a diagnosis, and finally present Mr AB with appropriate management options and agree on a management plan
- undertake opportunistic screening in view of BMI and BP; explore his health beliefs about weight and identify factors that might motivate him to lose weight

Brief to the patient – more about the patient

1. Profile:

- AB is a 34 year old single man
- he works in the accounts department of a local business
- he has been getting neck pain for the past 4 weeks

2. He is seeing the doctor today because:

- the pain is getting worse; it is localised to the right side of his neck at the back and does not radiate and he has no sensory changes or weakness in the arms. The pain gets worse during the day at work. It does not disturb his sleep and is not present on waking. He does not get the pain at weekends, even though he spends a lot of the time looking after his mother who is 'crippled with arthritis'.
- he has started taking ibuprofen and paracetamol at work to ease the pain
- his work is sedentary, checking account details on the computer
- he would like to be referred for physiotherapy as he believes his pain is due to sitting in front of a computer all day; he is happy to be given postural advice or exercises. He does not like taking tablets as he feels they only mask the problem and he is worried that doing so will result in long term damage to his neck.

3. Additional information:

- If the doctor asks specifically:
  - he has been moved to a different area of the office following a restructuring of the company. His new desk is small and the screen is set to one side, so he has to twist to look at it. He has an adjustable chair, but it is broken and the height is no longer adjustable. He is reluctant to make a fuss, because so many people lost their jobs in the restructuring. He would really like a letter from the doctor to give to his occupational health nurse suggesting that his workplace may be contributing to, or even causing, his neck pain.
  - he has no past history of neck or back pain
  - he is worried that arthritis is hereditary and that he is getting arthritis in his neck
- If the doctor asks about his weight:
  - he has put on more weight since last weighed; his mother is also obese, as was his father until he died of a heart attack age 55 years
  - he snores, but has no daytime somnolence
  - he follows no special diet; his mother likes 'good old-fashioned English food'. He buys sandwiches or crisps for lunch and always has sweets and chocolate in his office drawer. He drinks 1–2 cans of beer in the evenings. He despises smoking.

- o he knows he should lose weight, but finds it difficult to motivate himself, or to do it in isolation from his mother – he thinks eating is one of the few pleasures they both enjoy
- o he is concerned about his future health, especially as his father died of heart disease; if the doctor advises him in unambiguous terms that losing weight would benefit his health, he would address the problem
- if the doctor examines him:

System	Findings
General	Central obesity. Waist 40 inches (102 cm) Posture – rounded shoulders, protruding head BMI 36
Cardiovascular	Pulse 78 SR HS 1+2 nil No evidence of cardiomegaly or cardiac decompensation BP 150/94
Endocrine	No evidence of thyroid disease Urine negative for glucose
Cervical spine	Flexion – slightly reduced due to pain Extension – full Side flexion and rotation – slightly reduced to left, full to right Tender C5/6 on the left
Upper limb neurology	No sensory or motor loss Reflexes intact

Approach to be taken

A. Data gathering, examination and clinical assessment skills

1. *Define the clinical problem: clarify why the patient has presented today*
   The doctor:
   - reads the patient information provided prior to the consultation – notes the past history of lower limb fractures and raised BMI and BP
   - asks open questions to explore and clarify:
     o how Mr AB's neck pain affects him at home and at work
     o Mr AB's feelings about his weight and dieting
     o Mr AB's home circumstances
   - empathises with Mr AB over work and home situations
   - asks closed questions to exclude 'red flag' symptoms regarding his neck, metabolic causes for his obesity, and to assess his CVD risk
   - discovers AB's feelings about medication and his fear that arthritis is hereditary
   - uses internal summaries for each area to check that he has obtained the correct information

2. *Performs an appropriate physical or mental examination*
   - In this case, an examination is appropriate and should include:
     o posture – cervical spine movements and quick upper limb neurology check for sensation; the patient reports no neurological symptoms, so a detailed neurological examination is not necessary
     o cardiovascular – BP and BMI at minimum; calculate CVD risk
   - There is probably insufficient time to consider endocrine problems – hypothyroidism, Cushing's, diabetes, etc. These could be deferred to a follow-up appointment as he feels well.
   - Explain the purpose of examination in appropriate language.
   - The examination addresses the patient's ideas that his work is causing his pain and his concerns that he is developing neck arthritis.

B. Clinical management skills

3. *Make an appropriate working diagnosis*
   The doctor:
   - integrates information from the past and occupational histories, the pattern of pain, and the examination findings, to make a working diagnosis of postural neck pain
   - identifies that Mr AB has an increased CVD risk due to obesity, BP, lack of exercise, and family history

4. *Explain the problem to the patient using appropriate language*
   The doctor:
   - addresses Mr AB's agenda:
     - neck pain is probably due to the work-station set-up
     - Mr AB's weight and lifestyle are increasing his risk of CVD
   - provides information on posture and workplace set-up, CVD, and losing weight
   - explains the need to monitor Mr AB's BP and weight, and for him to modify his lifestyle
   - uses 'chunking and checking' to ensure accuracy of data collection and to check Mr AB's understanding at various stages throughout the consultation

5. *Provide holistic care and use resources effectively*
   The doctor:
   - practices evidence-based medicine – NICE obesity guidelines
   - discusses the role of the occupational nurse to assess his workplace
   - involves other members of the PHCT, such as the Practice Nurse, to give dietary advice and monitor Mr AB's weight and BP
   - understands socioeconomic/cultural background – job losses and having to look after his arthritic mother
   - demonstrates to Mr AB that the management of his problems share common features such as losing weight and increasing physical activity

6. *Prescribe appropriately*
   The doctor:
   - is aware of national and local guidelines (NICE guidelines on obesity and hypertension), and so dietary advice but not medication is indicated here
   - reassures Mr AB that the use of intermittent ibuprofen and paracetamol is appropriate to help when pain interferes with work. The doctor should check that there are no contraindications to NSAID use such as indigestion and asthma.
   - makes appropriate referral to physiotherapy for advice on self-management
   - arranges further checks of BP and weight
   - arranges dietary advice
   - provides a letter for Mr AB's occupational nurse

7. *Specify the conditions and interval for follow-up*
   The doctor:
   - signposts Mr AB to information on posture and exercise, and weight management and healthy eating
   - offers a follow-up appointment to check progress at work
   - offers a follow-up appointment with the Practice Nurse to monitor weight and BP
   - confirms understanding

C. Interpersonal skills: know and treat this patient

8. *Achieve rapport*
   The doctor:
   - listens attentively to Mr AB's concerns about his work and home situations
   - recognises verbal and non-verbal cues – Mr AB is reluctant to make a fuss at work as he is concerned about his job security
   - places problem in psychosocial context – how it may affect his ability to look after his mother
   - understands his request for physiotherapy and for a letter to his employers
   - discovers patient's health beliefs, e.g. that his workplace is contributing to his symptoms
   - addresses the patient's specific concerns and expectations

9. *Give the patient the opportunity to be involved in significant management decisions*
   The doctor:
   - encourages autonomy and opinions – provides patient with information and a letter to the occupational nurse to enable patient to tackle the cause of his neck pain
   - supports him in caring for his mother and explores whether additional help is required and would be acceptable to them

Debrief

This case could develop in several directions. The presenting complaint, neck pain, is relatively straightforward and the occupational cause should be identified readily. This should leave time to discuss Mr AB's weight problem and risks of CVD. However, there are other issues such as job insecurity and his mother's arthritis and increasing dependence on him that could deflect the doctor from completing the consultation in the available time.

Discuss how the doctor could, if needed, improve his performance. In particular, assess whether the doctor:
- identified that the neck pain was likely to be an occupational problem
- explored a range of management options with Mr AB – self-management exercises, posture advice, occupational nurse referral to name a few
- took the opportunity to talk about Mr AB's weight problem and the long-term effects of this on his health
- explored Mr AB's health beliefs and motivated him to lose weight and become more active
- arranged suitable investigation (work station assessment) and review

Revising data gathering

What questions could the doctor ask to discover the patient's ideas, concerns, expectations and health beliefs?
- Ideas: *"What do you think may have caused the neck pain?"*.
- Concerns: *"Are you concerned about your weight?"*.
- Expectations: *"It seems that your work may be causing your neck pain, shall we talk about how you might be able to improve things there?"*.
- Health beliefs:
  - *"Your father died of a heart attack at quite a young age, are you worried that this might affect you?"*.
  - *"You seem reluctant to take tablets for the neck pain, but if the pain is bad and affecting you, they can be useful, as correcting your posture and workplace may take some time to help things."*.

Once the doctor has gathered sufficient information, how could he summarise the problem for the patient?
- *"We have discussed a lot of issues today, and I would like to summarise back to you in case I've left out anything important or got anything wrong".*
- *"Your neck pain is most likely to be caused by your new work place; we have talked about how you might improve this at work and also about improving your posture. We have agreed that if things get worse, physiotherapy may ease the symptoms, but will not treat the cause, which you seem keen to tackle first".*

- *"We have discussed your risk of developing CVD given your family history, your increasing weight and BP. We have agreed to arrange some diet advice and support to lose weight and explore ways you can increase your physical activity".*

Test your theoretical knowledge

For each of the following statements, answer true (T) or false (F).

Regarding NICE guidance on management of obesity
1. BMI results should be interpreted with caution as they are not a direct measure of adiposity
2. Some of the following conditions must be met before bariatric surgery can be recommended – BMI >40; all other methods have failed after trials of at least 6 months; and the patient received intensive management in a specialist obesity service
3. Waist circumference gives information on risk of long-term health problems
4. Bioimpedance is recommended as a substitute for BMI because it is a quick and cheap way of accurately assessing adiposity
5. 5–10% weight loss has been shown to produce measurable health outcomes
6. Sibutramine is contraindicated in patients with high or poorly controlled blood pressure

Relevant literature

NICE (Dec 2006), *Obesity: guidance on the prevention, identification, assessment and management of overweight and obesity in adults and children*:
www.nice.org.uk/nicemedia/pdf/word/CG43NICEGuideline.doc

National Obesity Forum, Guidelines on the management of adult obesity and overweight in primary care:
www.nationalobesityforum.org.uk

Case 3 – Childhood eczema

Brief to the doctor

Mrs CC is a 36 year old woman who presents (without her son) asking for a repeat prescription for his eczema. She hands you a list of his medication.

Patient summary

Name	Darius C
Date of birth (Age)	2
Social and Family History	Only child, parents aged 36 and 33
Past medical history	Treated for a 'flare' 4 weeks ago with antibiotics and eumovate Seen in dermatology OPD 9 months ago – atopic eczema
Repeat medication	Doublebase thrice daily Aveeno at night Hydrocortisone as required or once daily for 7 days Oilatum Plus – use daily in bath

Tasks for the doctor

In this case, the tasks are to:
- clarify Mrs CC's concerns regarding her son's treatments
- review Darius' treatments, particularly efficacy and compliance
- prescribe appropriately

Brief to the patient – more about the patient

1. Profile:

- Mrs CC is a 36 year old woman who has returned to work (part-time) as an administrator
- married with 1 child, Darius, who has had eczema since infancy
- Mrs CC is worried about the severity of her son's eczema

2. She is seeing the doctor today because:

- she requires a repeat prescription of his medication
- she needs a set of emollients for nursery
- she recently attended a dinner party where one of the other guests, a health visitor, spoke to her about a new treatment, an 'anti-cancer' cream for eczema and she wants to talk to you about this
- she has not changed Darius' diet – should she?
- her mother-in-law is keen on taking Darius to see a local homeopath
- when asked about her application of the creams, she talks about applying the treatments conscientiously; she is concerned about nursery – they have only used one tube in three weeks and she uses a tube every week

3. Additional information:

- if the doctor discusses tacrolimus or pimecrolimus with her, she says she would like to read up about this before making a decision; she expects the doctor to signpost her to suitable information
- if Mrs CC feels comfortable with you, she volunteers her opinion on homeopathy – 'it is a load of drivel', however she would like your opinion; she also reveals her concern about her mother-in-law's interference, which she perceives as indirect criticism of her child raising

Approach to be taken

A. Data gathering, examination and clinical assessment skills

1. Define the clinical problem: clarify why the patient has presented today
The doctor:
- reads the patient information provided prior to the consultation
- asks open questions to explore how Darius is getting on with his treatment, the bathing and 'creaming' routine, his recovery from his recent flare, and what she thought helped him to improve
- empathises with her comments about how long the routine takes; this 'connection' with Mrs CC allows her to air her concerns regarding her suspicions that the nursery is not applying the emollients as diligently as she does at home
- asks closed questions to clarify details about the current appearance of the skin and which parts of the body are affected
- asks about current infection (weeping, pustules, malaise), facial eczema, sleep disturbance and nursery attendance, i.e. the doctor excludes red flags signalling the need for review or referral
- discovers Mrs CC's idea that homeopathy is 'drivel', her concern about nursery, her expectation for further information about tacrolimus / pimecrolimus and her health belief that diet may be linked to eczema

2. Performs an appropriate physical or mental examination
- In this case, an examination is not required.

B. Clinical management skills

3. Make an appropriate working diagnosis
- The doctor, based on the history, makes a working diagnosis of childhood atopic eczema; Mrs CC tells you that the dermatologists agreed with this diagnosis and initiated the current treatment regime.

4. Explain the problem to the patient using appropriate language
The doctor:
- having quickly established that Mrs CC is sensible and diligent in her application of the creams, addresses her agenda
- prescribes the medication and asks what she intends to do about nursery
- provides some information on the effectiveness of complementary and alternative (CAM) treatments – very little of it has good trial evidence and some may be harmful, for example, some Chinese herbal medicines for eczema have been found to contain dexamethasone
- explains that the health visitor may have been talking about tacrolimus or pimecrolimus; these immune suppressors may be useful for patients with moderate-to-severe disease, however, there is a theoretical increased risk

of developing skin cancer; they should be initiated by dermatologists or GPs with a special interest in dermatology, so it may be useful to discuss at the next OPD appointment
- advises Mrs CC that most children with atopic eczema do not have food allergy, and that exclusion diets rarely help. The importance of having a healthy balanced diet for growth and well-being is discussed.

5. *Provide holistic care and use resources effectively*
The doctor:
- practises evidence-based medicine
- is informed by national or local guidelines
- if Mrs CC is not overly concerned about the side-effects of steroid creams, then the doctor should not waste time addressing this issue – time is better spent addressing her concerns about diet and homeopathy

6. *Prescribe appropriately*
The doctor:
- is aware of national and local guidelines – www.nice.org.uk/nicemedia/pdf/CG057NICEGuideline.doc
- checks the patient's understanding of the medication and the amounts of medication required

7. *Specify the conditions and interval for follow-up*
The doctor:
- signposts Mrs CC to information on tacrolimus or pimecrolimus
- offers a follow-up appointment to discuss any issues arising from her reading; it would be useful to review Darius 'in the flesh' at this appointment to assess whether he meets criteria for initiation of these drugs

C. Interpersonal skills: know and treat this patient

8. *Achieve rapport*
The doctor:
- listens attentively to Mrs CC's concerns about nursery and her mother-in-law
- understands her request for information on alternative treatments
- displays empathy to the time-consuming routine and chronicity of the illness
- is non-judgemental about the patient's ideas on homeopathy and 'anti-cancer' creams
- addresses the patient's specific concerns and expectations

9. *Give the patient the opportunity to be involved in significant management decisions*
The doctor:
- encourages autonomy and opinions – provides her with information so she feels able to tackle treatment issues with nursery and her mother-in-law
- supports and congratulates her in caring for her son

Debrief

Discuss how the doctor could, if needed, improve his performance. In particular, assess whether the doctor:

- established rapport? If so, how?
- addressed Mrs CC's specific concerns? If so, how?
- discussed the evidence base for immune suppressors, exclusion diets and CAM?
- explained the risks and benefits of treatments in simple language?

If the consultation over-ran, did the doctor:

- repeat certain questions when taking the history?
- repeat some explanations?
- address issues the patient was not concerned about?

Revising data gathering

- What questions could the doctor ask to discover the patient's ideas, concerns, expectations and health beliefs?
- Ideas: *"I understand that your mother-in-law is keen on homeopathy. What is your view?"*
- Concerns: *"I agree that if applied as prescribed, nursery should have run out of cream much sooner. Are you concerned that they may not be applying the cream as directed?"*
- Expectations: *"It seems to me your recent discussion with the health visitor led to you to think about alternative treatments. I'll quickly outline the risks and benefits of these immune suppressor creams."*
- Health beliefs: *"You suspect that diet and eczema may be linked. Let's talk about this for a moment."*

Test your theoretical knowledge

For each of the following statements, answer true (T) or false (F).

1. A diagnosis of food allergy should be considered in children with atopic eczema who have reacted previously to a food with immediate symptoms.
2. A diagnosis of food allergy should be considered in infants with failure to thrive.
3. If leave-on emollients are prescribed in large quantities (250–500 g weekly), the child should be reviewed.
4. During flares affecting the face and neck, use moderate potency topical steroids for 3–5 days.
5. NICE recommends that health professionals review repeat prescriptions of products for children with atopic eczema at least twice a year.
6. Topical tacrolimus is recommended, within its licensed indications, as an option for the second-line treatment of moderate to severe atopic eczema, in adults and children aged 1 year and older, that has not been controlled by topical corticosteroids.

7. Healthcare professionals should offer a 1-month trial of a non-sedating antihistamine to children with severe atopic eczema.
8. Healthcare professionals should offer a 1-month trial of an age-appropriate sedating antihistamine to children aged 6 months or over during an acute flare of atopic eczema if sleep disturbance has a significant impact on the child or parents or carers.

Relevant literature

www.nice.org.uk/nicemedia/pdf/CG057NICEGuideline.doc

Case 4 – Tennis elbow

Brief to the doctor

Mrs CD is a 28 year old lady who presents with a right tennis elbow.

Patient summary

Name	CD
Date of birth (Age)	28
Social and family history	Married No children No recorded FH of CVD, DM
Past medical history	Seen 4 months ago: "*Repeat COCP. No problems.*"
	Seen 3 months ago: "*Persistent headaches – few weeks. Nil specific. Not unwell. Denies any worries. Diagnosis ?cause. Take OTC analgesia if reqd. Suggest watch and wait.*"
	Seen 1 month ago: "*Pain Rt shoulder/neck – 2 weeks. No cause identified. Full range of mvmt neck and shoulder. Declined analgesia. Offered physio but declined this as well.*"
Current medication	COCP

Investigations	3 months ago
BP	132/86
HR	84
	2 years ago – normal cervical smear
Smokes	<10/day

Tasks for the doctor

In this case, the tasks are to:
- assess the severity of Mrs CD's tennis elbow and agree a management plan
- respond to cues about her marriage and sensitively explore her satisfaction with her marriage and how she might try to improve the situation

Brief to the patient – more about the patient

1. Profile:

- Mrs CD is a 28 year old lady who is married to a leading local businessman who is 50 years old; they have a very comfortable lifestyle – large house, expensive cars and holidays
- she gave up her job as an art teacher when she married 4 years ago – she is frustrated that she is no longer working and gave up a profession
- she tries to occupy herself, but finds this difficult. She had to leave a local art group, which she really enjoyed, because her husband became very jealous that she was mixing with like-minded people, some of whom were her age and male. He has enrolled her in the tennis section at the golf club where he is a member and has bought her lessons there. He takes her to the club and plays golf with business acquaintances while she has lessons, then expects her to help entertain his guests over lunch.
- she feels she is used as a glamorous and vivacious 'trophy wife'
- she would like children, but her husband will not consider this as he feels children would distract him from work and prevent him enjoying his current lifestyle

2. She is seeing the doctor today because:

- her right elbow is sore after tennis; she thinks she can probably cope with it, but her husband has insisted she consult, in case it is something serious
- the elbow does not hurt at any other time. Her husband noticed it because she complained that her elbow hurt when driving him home after a business lunch. There has never been any swelling or loss of movement, nor any neurological symptoms. Her neck pain has gone.
- she does not expect or want any treatment. She would be very happy to be told to rest and avoid tennis for a while. She is not at all keen on medicines and prefers to use 'natural' remedies whenever possible.

3. Additional information:

- if the doctor asks specifically:
  - she feels very unhappy with her life and her marriage in particular – she regrets getting married and feels trapped
  - if pressed, she would accept that her presentations with persistent headaches, sore neck/shoulder and elbow pain are reflections of her unhappiness
- she would like the opportunity to talk about how she feels, but only after the doctor has given her enough time and information to enable her to reassure her husband that her elbow pain has been taken seriously. She will not raise

the subject, but will talk freely if the doctor raises the issue. She hopes that by dropping cues that she feels pressured into playing, and that she is not that bothered if told to rest completely, the doctor will suspect there is another matter she wishes to raise. However, if he asks her "*Is there anything else you want to talk about?*" without putting this into context, she will answer "*no*". She feels that the last doctor that saw her realised there was something else going on, but attempted to 'fob her off' by offering her physiotherapy.

- if asked:
  - she watches her weight very carefully as her husband criticises her if she gains any
  - she has trouble getting to sleep and wakes several times every night
  - she gets tearful easily and tries to avoid talking or thinking about her life because doing so upsets her
  - she has briefly considered suicide but dismissed the idea instantly as she wants to enjoy life not get out of it
  - she feels her parents would be very unsupportive as they disapproved of her marrying someone older and she thinks their attitude would be 'told you so' which she thinks would not be helpful; she is an only child
  - she has no close friends currently; however, she occasionally contacts an old boyfriend who is always very sympathetic and supportive – she occasionally thinks she should have married him
- if the doctor examines her:

System	Findings
Neck	Full range of movement Posture normal
Shoulder	Full range of movement Normal scapulothoracic rhythm
Elbow	Flexion/extension – full and pain-free Pronation/supination – full and pain-free No effusion Very slight tenderness on deep palpation over the lateral epicondyle No pain on resisted wrist dorsiflexion
Forearm	No swelling or tenderness
Neuro	No altered sensation or weakness; reflexes intact Neural tension tests negative

Approach to be taken

A. Data gathering, examination and clinical assessment skills

1. *Define the clinical problem: clarify why the patient has presented today*
   The doctor:
   - reads the patient information provided prior to the consultation, identifying several recent consultations for 'minor' problems
   - asks open questions to explore the presenting reason for her attendance (husband's concern), to clarify her symptoms (minor) and to ascertain how they affect her (minimally)
   - asks closed questions to exclude the neck as a cause of her pain
   - listens attentively and responds to cues such as her feeling pressurised into playing tennis
   - explores whether there are other issues she wishes to discuss using open and closed questions, silence and reference to previous attendances

2. *Performs an appropriate physical or mental examination*
   - In this case, a targeted examination is required – the minimally acceptable examination would be to exclude restricted elbow joint movement (flexion, extension, pronation and supination) and localised swelling or tenderness
   - the examination should address the patient's (and her husband's) concerns
   - a 'gold standard' examination would include neck and shoulder movements and systematic examination of the upper limb

B. Clinical management skills

3. *Make an appropriate working diagnosis*
   The doctor:
   - integrates information from previous consultations, questions about her presenting complaint, cues and questions about her happiness
   - identifies and explores, by using a patient-centred approach, the real reason for the patient's attendance
   - makes a working diagnosis of mild tennis elbow and underlying marital unhappiness

4. *Explain the problem to the patient using appropriate language*
   The doctor:
   - having quickly established that this was a case of mild tennis elbow, gives appropriate management advice – rest from tennis
   - agrees with the patient that medication and referral for physiotherapy are not appropriate
   - provides some information on the effectiveness of complementary and alternative (CAM) treatments – acupuncture/dry needling, and exercises and self-management techniques may help

5. *Provide holistic care and use resources effectively*
The doctor:
- does not make an unnecessary physiotherapy referral or prescribe analgesia
- by exploring the socioeconomic/cultural background, is likely to discover the real reason for the attendance

6. *Prescribe appropriately*
The doctor:
- agrees not to prescribe any medication
- explores a range of management strategies to deal with her unhappiness – how she might raise her frustration at no longer working and having to be a 'trophy wife' with her husband

7. *Specify the conditions and interval for follow-up*
The doctor:
- offers a follow-up to explore her feelings about her marriage

C. Interpersonal skills: know and treat this patient

8. *Achieve rapport*
The doctor:
- listens attentively to Mrs CD's explanations of her symptoms
- explores and clarifies her symptoms and feelings
- recognises verbal and non-verbal cues – not being concerned about having to rest from tennis
- sensitively explores Mrs CD's unhappiness with her marriage and frustration with her lifestyle
- places the problem in psychosocial context – her husband pressurising her to play tennis
- discovers the patient's health beliefs and understands her reluctance to have medication

9. *Give the patient the opportunity to be involved in significant management decisions*
The doctor:
- actively confirms patient's understanding of the problem, i.e. that her tennis elbow is mild and requires no active treatment
- supports and empathises with her marital unhappiness
- explores various strategies for improving her lifestyle and hence happiness

Debrief

The presenting symptom, tennis elbow, is minor and the real issue in this consultation is picking up the patient's cues about her marriage and then exploring this issue.

Discuss how the doctor could, if needed, improve his performance. In particular, assess how the doctor:

- established rapport with Mrs CD
- identified the underlying issue
- explored strategies Mrs CD might employ to raise or address her unhappiness

Revising data gathering

What questions could the doctor ask to discover the patient's ideas, concerns, expectations and health beliefs?

- Ideas: *"Are you happy that I have excluded a serious problem with your elbow?"*
- Concerns: *"You said that your husband has made you come today, why do you think he has done that?"*
- Expectations: *"It seems to me that the last few times you have come here you have had problems that you didn't want any treatment for. Sometimes that happens when people are worried about something else and so I wonder if there is another problem, perhaps a personal one, that you would like to discuss?"*
- Health beliefs: *"I see you were not keen on painkillers before, is that because you don't like taking medicines?"*

Once the doctor has gathered sufficient information, how could he summarise the problem for the patient?

- *"Your elbow pain does not seem to interfere with you that much and my examination is pretty normal"*

If the consultation over-ran, did the doctor:

- allow the patient to repeat herself or not offer useful information?
- not understand why the patient had attended?
- not pick up the patient's cues?
- find it difficult discussing personal issues and feelings with the patient?
- spend too much time data gathering and not enough time listening?
- fail to organise and structure the consultation appropriately?

Test your theoretical knowledge

For each of the following statements, answer true (T) or false (F).

Regarding tennis elbow
1. It is an overuse injury involving the flexor muscle origin on the lateral epicondylar region of the humerus
2. Pain may radiate into the forearm

3. 90% or more of cases respond to conservative management
4. Corticosteroid injections give rapid and lasting relief
5. Extracorporeal shock wave treatment has been shown to be beneficial
6. Topical nitric oxide (by applying GTN patches) may improve outcome
7. The current fashion for oversized racquets with high string tension increases the risk of developing tennis elbow

Relevant literature

Bisset L, Paungmail A, Vicenzino B, *et al.* (2005) A systematic review and meta-analysis of clinical trials on physical interventions for lateral epicondylalagia. *Br J Sports Med,* **39**: 411–422.

Paoloni JA, Appleyard RC, Nelson J, *et al.* (2003) Topical nitric oxide application in the treatment of chronic extensor tendinosis at the elbow: a randomised, double-blinded, placebo-controlled clinical trial. *Am J Sports Med,* **31**: 915–920.

Smidt N, van der Windt D, Assendelft W, *et al.* (2002) Corticosteroid injections, a physiotherapy, or wait-and-see policy for lateral epicondylitis: a randomised controlled trial. *Lancet,* **359**: 657–662.

Waugh EJ, Jaglal SB, Davis AM (2004) Computer use associated with poor long-term prognosis of conservatively managed lateral epicondylalgia. *J Orthop Sports Phys Ther,* **34**: 770–780.

Case 5 – Ankle injury

Brief to the doctor

Mr TP is a 22 year old man who presents with a sore ankle (right). He walks into your surgery on crutches. He is due to leave for Ghana in 5 weeks as part of a VSO team.

Patient summary

Name	TP
Date of birth (Age)	22
Social and Family History	Unmarried
Past medical history	Tonsillitis 3 years ago Insomnia 6 years ago
Current medication	None
Blood tests	Tests were done 4 months ago (VSO medical)
BMI	27
BP	128/68

Tasks for the doctor

In this case, the tasks are to:
- assess how the ankle injury impacts on his life
- provide him with information about healing times
- help him to reach a decision about physiotherapy and his fitness to undertake volunteer work in a remote area

Brief to the patient – more about the patient

1. Profile:

- Mr TP is a 22 year old man
- unmarried and not currently in a relationship
- works with his father in the building trade undertaking barn conversions and building renovations
- due to start a 3-month VSO placement in Ghana in 5 weeks
- injured his ankle during a football game with his mates 7 days ago; attended A&E where an X-ray ruled out an ankle fracture – he was told to take analgesia and to see his GP for further treatment
- in the week since the injury, he has mobilised well on crutches, is now weight-bearing on the ankle and takes one 400 mg ibuprofen thrice daily

2. He is seeing the doctor today because:

- the A&E doctor told him he didn't have a fracture but didn't give any advice about mobilizing or running
- the box of tablets he was given says he should take one tablet three times a day after meals – for how long should he continue with the tablets?
- he has tried putting weight through the ankle and has walked from his bed to the toilet without crutches – although it was painful (5/10), it was bearable
- what should he do about crutches; when can he start running again; does he need physiotherapy?
- he would like to know if his ankle will be healed within 5 weeks; he is worried about letting his VSO team members down if he needs extra help or if he cannot carry out certain physical tasks such as helping to build a water pipe; also, in Ghana, he will be living in a remote rural area some distance from medical care
- when he contacted VSO for advice, they advised him to consult his GP first
- he does not have private health insurance; if you advise him to pay to see a physiotherapist, he is happy to do so, especially if you think physiotherapy can get his ankle strong again for his Ghana trip
- if the doctor offers him a 'wait and see' policy, he wants to know what he should tell VSO
- if the doctor offers him an NHS physiotherapy referral, he wants to know the likelihood of being seen within 5 weeks
- by the way, he has season tickets to the local football club (worth approximately £550); his parents don't go to games, so would the doctor like the tickets? He is grateful to the practice for organising his VSO medical at short notice and for waiving their fee.

Approach to be taken

A. Data gathering, examination and clinical assessment skills

1. *Define the clinical problem: clarify why the patient has presented today*
   The doctor:
   - notes, from the medical record, that Mr TP had a VSO medical 4 months ago
   - detects a non-verbal cue – Mr TP walks in on crutches; on questioning the reason for the crutches, the doctor obtains a history of the ankle injury and the hospital treatment
   - asks open questions to explore what specifically about the ankle injury brings him to the surgery today, i.e. the doctor explores his expectations and concerns
   - asks focused and closed questions to clarify details of the pain, analgesia, and ability to mobilize
   - elicits how the problem affects Mr TP and discovers his concerns about being fit to travel to Ghana in 5 weeks as part of a VSO team
   - explores his health beliefs that physiotherapy would lead to quicker healing
   - summarises the problem: as regards your ankle sprain, you are consulting today for advice on painkillers, when to restart running, and whether you should go to Ghana in 5 weeks – have I understood you correctly?

2. *Perform an appropriate physical or mental examination*
   - An examination of the ankle is unlikely to be needed given the history of improvements (in pain and mobility) and the fact that the patient does not have specific concerns warranting physical reassessment.

B. Clinical management skills

3. *Make an appropriate working diagnosis*
   The doctor:
   - recognises from the history that the patient is describing a typical grade 2 ankle sprain (www.cks.nhs.uk/sprains_and_strains#-323177)
   - recognises that the ankle injury is healing as it should be (i.e. following the expected pattern of illness)

4. *Explain the problem to the patient using appropriate language*
   The doctor:
   - is patient-centred – uses the patient's ideas on mobilizing (without crutches) as pain allows, reducing NSAIDs and perhaps changing to analgesics, and starting rehabilitation of the ankle (explaining that running may not be the best way to achieve ankle strength and stability – www.cks.library.nhs.uk/sprains_and_strains/in_depth/management_issues)

- uses the patient's beliefs regarding physiotherapy – explains that initial physiotherapy treatment with ultrasound or infrared attempts to reduce swelling and pain, and that later rehabilitation teaches stretching and strengthening exercises to prevent re-injury
- provides information on healing times: grade 2 sprains – people usually start walking on the ankle after 2 days of rest; the swelling goes down after 7–10 days; people in physically demanding jobs may take a few weeks to return to work and people may not be able to take part in sport for a few months
- addresses the patient's concerns and expectations – explores the risks and benefits of postponing the VSO trip until the ankle has regained full strength (this may take a few months) versus going to Ghana where walking on uneven ground may put an incompletely healed ankle at risk of re-injury

5. *Provide holistic care and use resources effectively*
The doctor:
- may, after discussion with the patient, refer to physiotherapy (NHS or private based on his preference)
- practises evidence-based medicine
- is informed by national or local guidelines – www.cks.library.nhs.uk/ sprains_and_strains/in_summary

6. *Prescribe appropriately*
The doctor:
- is aware of national and local guidelines
- chooses cost-effective medication (paracetamol rather than codeine; ibuprofen rather than alternative NSAIDs)
- checks the patient's understanding of the medication and warns the patient about potential side effects

7. *Specify the conditions and interval for follow-up*
- The doctor outlines expected healing times and advises the patient to return for re-assessment if he does not heal as predicted

C. Interpersonal skills: know and treat this patient

8. *Achieve rapport*
The doctor:
- understands how important the VSO trip is to him and displays empathy with his bad luck
- addresses the patient's specific concerns (about rehabilitation) and his expectations regarding VSO
- thanks the patient for his offer of the football tickets, which raises an ethical issue: does the offer affect the doctor's decision-making in any way; how does the doctor politely refuse the gift; if the gift is accepted, does the

doctor explain to Mr TP the new stipulation in the GP contract that GPs keep a register of gifts with a value over £100?

9. *Give the patient the opportunity to be involved in significant management decisions*
The doctor:
- shares his thoughts on healing times, the value of rehabilitation and involves the patient in decisions
- encourages autonomy and opinions – asks Mr TP questions that allow him to evaluate the benefits and risks of going to Ghana in 5 weeks, thus facilitating his decision-making

Debrief

Discuss how the doctor could, if needed, improve his performance. In particular, assess whether the doctor:

- understood the reason for the patient's attendance today or whether he made assumptions regarding the patient's agenda? If so, what questions or explanations did the doctor use that led him down this incorrect track?
- asked questions that facilitated Mr TP's decision-making or did the doctor make decisions for him?
- deal with the gift ethically and sensitively?

If the consultation over-ran:

- did the doctor repeat his questions or explanations?
- perform any unnecessary examinations?
- get embarrassed or flummoxed by the gift?

Revising data gathering

What questions could the doctor ask to discover the patient's ideas, concerns, expectations and health beliefs?

- Ideas: *"I understand that you want your ankle to heal as fast as possible. Did you have any ideas on how we could achieve this?"*
- Concerns: *"What is your ankle injury preventing you from doing, at work or socially? Is there anything in particular about your fitness that concerns you?"*
- Expectations: *"When you came into surgery today, what is it that you hoped I would do for you?"*
- Health beliefs: *"Am I right in thinking that you believe the ankle will heal faster with physiotherapy? Let's talk about what improves ankle healing in the short and long term."*

Test your theoretical knowledge

For each of the following statements, answer true (T) or false (F).
1. Rest sprained ankles for 24 hours, after which active movement should be encouraged.
2. Place a bag of ice on to the swollen ankle for 20 minutes, allowing 2 hours in between applications for re-warming.
3. Advise patients to improve balance by walking with the eyes shut, once the pain has settled.
4. Ibuprofen, prescribed to patients with cardiovascular disease, may reduce the cardiovascular protective effect of low-dose aspirin.
5. More than 75% of ankle injuries are ankle fractures.

Relevant literature

www.cks.library.nhs.uk/sprains_and_strains/view_whole_guidance

Case 6 – MRI result – back pain

Brief to the doctor

Mr EF, age 42, wishes to discuss the treatment options for his back following a recent MRI scan organised by the hospital orthopaedic department. He has previously been seeing one of your partners who is now on maternity leave.

Patient summary

Name	EF
Date of birth (Age)	42
Past medical history	1 year ago – GP notes:*"LBP with Rt L5 pain and paraesthesia – 3 months. Private physio and osteopath have not helped. Ibuprofen and Co-codamol 30/500 (prescribed by dental colleague) not helped. V stiff L spine. SLR 30 on Rt, 90 on Lt. Absent Ankle Jerk. Letter from physio suggesting referral. Refer Orthopaedics"*
	9 months ago – Letter from Specialist Physio Clinic: *"5 months LBP with L5 sciatica. No red flags. Has only had manipulative treatment in private sector, for outpatient physio."*
	7 months ago – GP notes: *"Hospital physio referred him for more physio – v unhappy. Getting worse. Interfering with ability to work, considering having to reduce workload, partners at work not happy with him. Wants to see orthopaedic consultant not physio. Letter to consultant requesting he review patient."*
	5 months ago – Consultant letter: *"Thank you for asking me to see Mr EF. I think the time has come to establish the cause of his back and leg pain and have arranged an MRI. I have warned him that there is likely to be a wait for this. I will see him when he has had the scan to discuss treatment options."*
	2 weeks ago – MRI result: *"Reduced signal L4/5 and L5/S1 discs. There is a large Rt sided disc protrusion compressing the L5 root."*

Current medication   Ibuprofen 400 mg 1 tab 3 or 4 times daily with food
          Co-codamol 30/500 2 tabs 4 times daily as required

Tasks for the doctor

In this case, the tasks are to:

- explain the MRI result and treatment options to Mr EF
- explore his concerns about treatments and their long and short-term effects on his health and work (expectations)
- support and explore his disappointment with the quality of care he has received from the hospital

Brief to the patient – more about the patient

1. Profile:

- 42 year old partner in a local private dental practice and is married with 2 children aged 10 and 8 years
- he developed low back pain and right sciatica 15 months ago and initially saw an osteopath and then a physiotherapist privately, but did not respond to treatment. His physiotherapist advised that he needed a scan and possibly an operation. He therefore attended his GP and was referred to the orthopaedic department at the local hospital for an MRI.
- he was seen by a specialist physiotherapist at the hospital who was very critical of the treatment he had received from both the osteopath and from the physiotherapist. He was told there was no indication for an urgent scan and that he should attend the hospital outpatient physiotherapy department for 'proper' physiotherapy.
- he was very unhappy at not being seen by a consultant as he feels that it was discourteous to a fellow health practitioner; he was not happy with the clinic recommendations, but did not want to make a fuss and so complied with the recommendations
- attending physiotherapy outpatients was very disruptive to his practice as the department only offered appointments during the working day. He had already reduced his workload with his partners' agreement, but he sensed that they were getting disgruntled with his reduced presence and contribution to the practice.
- his symptoms did not respond to outpatient physiotherapy and so he saw his GP again and requested a consultant appointment. When he saw the consultant, he was immediately referred for an MRI scan.

2. He is seeing the doctor today because:

- he had the scan 2 weeks ago and would like to know the result
- he has an outpatient appointment in 6 weeks, and would like to discuss what treatments he is likely to be offered by the consultant
- he is concerned that he may never return to full working ability again, even after a back operation
- he wonders whether he would have got better and quicker treatment if he had been seen privately or if he had the MRI earlier
- if there is time, he would like to discuss making a complaint about the treatment he has received at the hospital, particularly the delay in getting the MRI

3. Additional information:

- if the doctor asks specifically:
  - he has constant back and leg pain and is kept awake by pain and so sleeps only fitfully

- o he feels that his right leg is getting weak and the pins and needles are now constant. Coughing, sneezing and straining produce leg pain. He has no problems with bowel or bladder control and no perineal numbness. His weight is stable.
  - o his pain is made worse by bending or twisting, which he has to do frequently at work
  - o he is a keen runner but has not been able to run since his back pain started
  - o the constant pain and lack of sleep are making him grumpy and short-tempered; while he manages to control this at work, if pressed, he has taken it out on his wife and children, but has never been violent.
- he is concerned that his business partners could ask him to leave the partnership or reduce his share of the profits due to his reduced workload. With 2 children at private school, he cannot afford to reduce his income.
- he believes that an operation is indicated and that if the hospital had listened to his GP and private physiotherapist, he could have had the operation by now and hence not be worrying about the effects on work, as well as sparing him and his family from the effects of his worsening symptoms
- he does not want an epidural and will refuse a referral to the Pain Clinic
- he trusts his GPs as they have always given him honest, sensible and unbiased advice
- he does not like to make a fuss and looks to his GP to be his advocate, but feels he should be treated as a priority due to the adverse effect of his problem on work and home
- he has some savings and has discussed with his wife whether to use these to fund an operation privately in order to get it done quickly
- if the doctor examines him:

System	Findings
General	Walks slowly and sits with difficulty Looks tired and drawn
Lumbar spine	Flattened lordosis Flexion-fingertips to top of patella Extension – nil Side flexion – reduced to the right more than to the left Tender palpation L4/5 and L5/S1 Spasm and tenderness of paraspinal muscles
Neurology	SLR 70 left with some cross pain, 20 right Slump test pos. on right Femoral stretch negative bilaterally Absent sensation L5 (right) Weak big toe extension and foot eversion (right) Absent ankle jerk (right)

Approach to be taken

A. Data gathering, examination and clinical assessment skills

1. Define the clinical problem: clarify why the patient has presented today
The doctor:
- reads the patient information provided prior to the consultation
- uses a well organised approach to gather information
- asks open questions to explore how Mr EF is getting on in terms of symptoms and how they are affecting his life – *"How is all this affecting you at work and home?"*
- asks closed questions to clarify details about level of pain, weakness and paraesthesia, and to exclude cauda equina symptoms
- discovers Mr EF's belief that an operation is required and that this should be done as soon as possible
- explores and clarifies the impact his symptoms are having on his home life

2. Performs an appropriate physical or mental examination
- In this case, an examination is required as Mr EF has indicated that his symptoms have worsened, in particular that he has developed weakness.
- A targeted examination should be made concentrating on lower limb neurology.

B. Clinical management skills

3. Make an appropriate working diagnosis
- The doctor integrates information from the history, scan result and examination, and makes a working diagnosis of L5 nerve root compression due to prolapsed lumbar intervertebral disc.

4. Explain the problem to the patient using appropriate language
The doctor:
- uses the patient's ideas and beliefs and explains the MRI result and indicates that the consultant is most likely to offer an operation – *"Do you know much about back operations?"*
- explains the natural history of prolapsed discs
- outlines the various options available while not pre-empting the consultant's opinion – operation, epidural, pain clinic
- provides some information on recovery times and functional outcomes from operations in order to address the patient's concerns
- reviews the effectiveness, or not, of Mr EF's current analgesia
- checks understanding – *"Does my explanation make sense? Is there anything else you would like to ask?"*

5. *Provide holistic care and use resources effectively*
The doctor:
- practises evidence-based medicine
- is informed by national or local guidelines
- understands and explores the socioeconomic background – effects on work and home life

6. *Prescribe appropriately*
The doctor:
- reviews Mr EF's current analgesia regimen and prescribes tramadol
- checks the patient's understanding of the medication and the amounts of medication required
- discovers whether Mr EF would like to elect for private treatment at this point in time or wait to see the outcome of the outpatient appointment
- decides whether to discuss the urgency of the case with the consultant based on the history and examination findings, but also in view of the patient's dissatisfaction with the treatment received thus far

7. *Specify the conditions and interval for follow-up*
- The doctor ensures Mr EF is aware of the 'red flag symptoms' – safety netting

C. Interpersonal skills: know and treat this patient

8. *Achieve rapport*
The doctor:
- listens attentively to Mr EF's description of his symptoms and their effect on work and home
- may use verbal and non-verbal cues to clarify the degree of Mr EF's disability: *"You seem to have difficulty moving around, is that causing you any problems?"*
- places problem in a psychosocial context – how it affects patient/family
- understands his request for information on recovery and success of treatments
- displays empathy – *"How are you coping?"*
- explores patient's health ideas, concerns and expectations
- is understanding but non-judgemental about the advice and opinion Mr EF was given in his initial hospital appointment; gives advice about making a complaint if Mr EF requests this
- supports Mr EF's efforts to continue working and remain active

9. *Give the patient the opportunity to be involved in significant management decisions*
The doctor:
- actively confirms the patient's understanding of the problem
- shares thoughts/involves patient in deciding how to progress management: *"There are a number of options here... Which of these do you prefer?"*

Debrief

Discuss how the doctor could, if needed, improve his performance. In particular, assess whether the doctor:
- achieved rapport
- dealt with Mr EF's unhappiness with aspects of his treatment by the hospital
- addressed Mr EF's concerns about the impact on his ability to work both in the short and the long term

If the consultation over-ran, did the doctor:
- manage the time available appropriately and in a structured and organised way?
- concentrate on addressing the issues Mr EF was most concerned about (impact on work and family life) or get bogged-down dealing with some aspects of the case (dissatisfaction with the hopsital)?

Revising data gathering

What questions could the doctor ask to discover the patient's ideas, concerns, expectations and health beliefs?
- Ideas: *"Now the scan has confirmed the clinical diagnosis of a disc prolapse, what treatment do you think the consultant is likely to recommend?".*
- Concerns: *"You have told me that you feel under pressure from your partners because you have had to reduce your workload; how do you think they are going to feel if you have to have an operation?".*
- Expectations: *"It seems to me that you believe you need an operation, would you like me to outline the basic options available to you?".*
- Health beliefs: *"You seem concerned that your symptoms may not recover after an operation, would you like to discuss the success rates of operations with myself or the consultant?".*

Test your theoretical knowledge

For each of the following statements, answer true (T) or false (F):
1. The reported lifetime prevalence of back pain varies between 49 and 70%
2. Rare causes of sciatica include tumours and lumbar stenosis
3. Straight leg raising (Lasègue's sign) is a very sensitive and specific test
4. Computed tomography and magnetic resonance imaging are equally accurate at diagnosing lumbar disc herniation
5. Surgical discectomy provides faster relief from acute sciatica than conservative management

Relevant literature

Gibson JN, Waddell G. (2007) Surgical interventions for lumbar disc prolapse. *Cochrane Database Syst Rev,* **1**: CD001350.

Carragee EJ. (2005) The surgical treatment of disc degeneration: is the race not to be too swift? *Spine,* **5**: 587–588.

Koes BW, van Tulder MW, Peul WC. (2007) Diagnosis and treatment of sciatica. *BMJ,* **334:** 1313–1317.

www.lowbackpain.tv

Case 7 - Foot pain

Brief to the doctor

Mr SF is a 37 year old man who presents with a 4-day history of worsening foot pain (right). He requests analgesia. He had blood tests done 5 months ago and was advised to make lifestyle changes.

Patient summary

Name	SF
Date of birth (Age)	37
Social and Family History	Married, two children
	Dad fatal MI aged 69
Past medical history	Hypercholesterolaemia (5 months ago)
	Morton's neuroma 2nd left toe (1 year ago)
	Gout (2 years ago)
Current medication	None

Blood tests Tests were done 5 months ago

Plasma fasting glucose	5.8 mmol/l (3.65–5.5)
Fasting cholesterol	7.2 mmol/l
Fasting HDL cholesterol	0.8 mmol/l (0.8–1.8)
Total cholesterol:HDL	9
TSH	1.89 (0.35–5.5)
Alkaline phosphatase	156 IU/l (95–280)
Total bilirubin	14 µmol/l (3–17)
Albumin	46 g/l (35–50)
Creatinine level	99 µmol/l (70–150)
BMI	34
BP	141/86
Framingham	12%
Plasma urate (2 years ago)	467 (210–480)

Tasks for the doctor

In this case, the tasks are to:
- advise Mr SF on analgesia and prescribe appropriately
- talk to Mr SF about his lifestyle changes
- arrange suitable follow-up

Brief to the patient - more about the patient

1. Profile:

- Mr SF is a 37 year old man
- married with 2 young children
- he works as an administrator for a logistics company, mainly office-based
- his dad died 6 months ago of a fatal MI; this prompted him to see his GP for a health check – his cholesterol was high
- he was told to reduce his cholesterol by changing his diet, taking more exercise and losing weight; he found dieting difficult; hence 2 weeks ago, he started a Slighter Lite programme of pre-prepared meals
- he had severe foot pain 2 years ago; he was told it was gout, but the follow-up blood test did not show a raised plasma urate so he is confused about the original diagnosis

2. He is seeing the doctor today because:

- he has severe pain in his right foot – he started taking ibuprofen 400 mg thrice daily because he suspected gout, but the foot remains painful; he wants stronger analgesia
- he is confused by the plasma urate test result – does he have gout even if the urate level was normal?
- he feels frustrated as the foot pain has interrupted his exercise programme; he finds dieting difficult as it is and feels angry with this further set-back to his weight loss programme
- if questioned about the Slighter Lite programme, he tells you it is a very low calorie, low carbohydrate diet; he is getting on well with it, having lost 9 kg in 2 weeks
- he is worried about his raised cholesterol because of his dad's fatal MI 6 months ago.
- he expects the doctor to give him advice about gout, to prescribe analgesia, to advise him on when to repeat his blood tests, and to specify which tests are needed and why

Approach to be taken

A. Data gathering, examination and clinical assessment skills

1. *Define the clinical problem: clarify why the patient has presented today*
   The doctor:
   - makes use of the medical records provided; notices the family history, raised cholesterol, history of gout with a normal serum urate from 2 years ago
   - sees that Mr SF limps in and has a facial expression of pain; he responds to this non-verbal cue immediately, with an appropriate opening sentence such as *"You look as if you have a sore foot"*.
   - asks open questions, such as *"How can I help you today?"* to explore the reasons for Mr SF's presentation today
   - asks closed questions, such as *"On a scale of 1–10, how severe is the pain?"* and *"Where exactly is the pain?"* to clarify details of the foot pain
   - works through a diagnostic sieve to exclude other causes of foot pain (such as trauma or Morton's neuroma) and excludes red flags (septic arthritis or rheumatoid arthritis) by asking *"Are you unwell in yourself? Any temperature symptoms or general body aches?"*
   - elicits how the problem is affecting the patient, his family, or his work: *"Were you able to work with this? How are you managing at home?"*
   - discovers Mr SF's ideas: *"I see from your notes you had gout 2 years ago. Do you think this might be gout?"*
   - discovers Mr SF's concerns: *"What are your concerns about what has happened to you?"*
   - discovers Mr SF's expectations: *"By the end of this consultation, what questions would you like to have had answered?"*
   - discovers Mr SF's health beliefs: *"Am I right in thinking that you doubt the diagnosis of gout because the blood test 2 years ago was normal?"*
   - summarises the problem: *"This sounds like gout, but I would like to examine you. Is that OK?"*

2. *Perform an appropriate physical or mental examination*
   The doctor:
   - performs an appropriate physical examination: number of joints affected, erythema, swelling, tenderness and range of motion; if there is diagnostic doubt, takes the patient's temperature, and explains why the examination is being done
   - performs the examination slickly and with sensitivity
   - explains the examination findings in appropriate language, for example, *"One joint is affected, where the big toe meets the instep; it is red, swollen, warm and painful to touch and move; this is typical of gout"*

B. Clinical management skills

3. *Make an appropriate working diagnosis*
   The doctor:
   - integrates information: recognises conditions associated with gout, such as obesity and hypercholesterolaemia
   - on the basis of probability, makes a clinically sound working diagnosis: understands that serum urate measured during the acute attack may be normal; serum urate should be measured 4–6 weeks after the acute attack has resolved

4. *Explain the problem to the patient using appropriate language*
   The doctor:
   - is patient-centred – uses the patient's ideas and beliefs: *"I can understand why the normal blood test made you doubt the diagnosis of gout, but if the test was done in the middle of the attack, it could be misleading; this looks like gout and we are better off doing the test for gout 6 weeks after this episode settles"*
   - paces the explanation appropriately – *"How do you feel about us sorting the pain out now and doing the blood tests later?"*
   - provides information in adequate chunks and checks understanding at each step – *"Did you know that a diet with lots of meat and alcohol can cause gout?"*; after Mr SF responds, the doctor could then say *"Actually, crash dieting with high protein / low carb. diets can also precipitate gout"*
   - addresses the patient's concerns about his difficulty in losing weight – *"Congratulations on losing 9 kg; this shows motivation and hard work, but do you think this type of eating is sustainable? Could you make smaller changes that you could incorporate into your daily routine?"*
   - addresses the patient's expectations – prescribes an NSAID to be used until 48 hours after the acute attack has resolved – and gives the patient the option: does he want a particular tablet he's used successfully in the past?
   - summarises the problem – *"This looks like gout, which we'll treat using an anti-inflammatory tablet. I'll let you think about whether you want to stop the Slighter Lite diet, but I think it's probably precipitated this attack. We'll confirm if it's gout with a blood test in 6 weeks. It may be useful to repeat your cholesterol and fasting glucose tests at the same time."*
   - actively confirms the patient's understanding of the problem – *"We've discussed quite a lot today. So that I know I've explained properly, could you summarise the plan for me?"*

5. *Provide holistic care and use resources effectively*
   The doctor:
   - makes balanced plans which are either doctor or patient-centred as appropriate – negotiates analgesia, and advises on diet and alcohol intake without hectoring or preaching to the patient

- refers appropriately to the Primary Health Care Team (such as the phlebotomist) and other agencies (such as a dietician) if needed
- practises evidence-based medicine and is informed by national or local guidelines, such as: www.cks.nhs.uk/gout/management/quick_answers/scenario_acute_gout

6. *Prescribe appropriately*
The doctor:
- chooses cost-effective medication, such as diclofenac, indometacin or naproxen, with or without paracetamol and codeine
- discusses medication side effects
- checks the patient's understanding of the medication

7. *Specify the conditions and interval for follow-up*
The doctor:
- safety-nets appropriately: *"If you take the tablets regularly and there is no improvement in the pain within 3 days, could you come back to see me?"*

C. Interpersonal skills: know and treat this patient

8. *Achieve rapport*
The doctor:
- listens attentively, picking up the patient's pain, frustration and uncertainty about the diagnosis, and displays empathy to any adverse psychosocial consequences – *"I can see how you thought this diet would be the solution"*
- uses the patient's ideas about the blood test in his explanations
- addresses the patient's specific concerns about weight management and expectations for acute treatment with appropriate NSAIDs / analgesia

9. *Give the patient the opportunity to be involved in significant management decisions*
The doctor:
- shares thoughts and involves the patient in decisions – *"Any ideas about which painkillers work best for you?"*
- negotiates with the patient – *"I think your low carb. diet may be precipitating this. What do you think? Where can you find more information about the side-effects of this diet?"*
- offers choices or various treatment options – *"I can start with a very potent NSAID and step down, or I could start with a potent one and if it doesn't work, you could combine it with paracetamol. Which option would you prefer?"*
- encourages autonomy and opinions – *"Have a think and decide how you want to manage your weight long term"*

Debrief

Discuss how the doctor could, if needed, improve his performance. In particular, assess whether the doctor:

- established good rapport? If so, which behaviour created rapport? Which statements were particularly useful in achieving rapport?
- presented the patient with appropriate treatment options? Did the doctor risk-assess appropriately prior to prescribing? Did the doctor give appropriate lifestyle advice?
- signposted appropriately? For example, prior to examining, did he ask, *"I'd like to examine you now, is that OK?"*
- summarised appropriately? *"This looks like gout, which we'll treat using an anti-inflammatory tablet. I'll let you think about whether you want to stop the Slighter Lite diet, but I think it's probably precipitated this attack. We'll confirm if it's gout with a blood test in 6 weeks. It may be useful to repeat your cholesterol and fasting glucose tests at the same time."*

If the consultation over-ran:

- was the doctor systematic in his history taking? Did he repeat questions? Did he allow the patient to ramble on uninterrupted?
- were the doctor's explanations simple and non-judgemental?

Revising data gathering

What questions could the doctor ask to discover the patient's ideas, concerns, expectations and health beliefs?

- Ideas: *"What do you think has caused this attack of foot pain?"*
- Concerns: *"Was there anything you were particularly worried about?"*
- Expectations: *"Am I right in thinking you'd like some strong painkillers?"*
- Health beliefs: *"It seems to me that you are slightly confused by the normal blood test result you had two years ago. Shall we discuss how gout is diagnosed in more detail?"*

Test your theoretical knowledge

For each of the following statements, answer true (T) or false (F).

1. Advise patients with gout to avoid purine-rich foods, such as bananas, chocolate and tuna.
2. Consider prophylactic medication with colchicine if a person is having two or more attacks of gout in a year.
3. Seek specialist advice if gout occurs during pregnancy.
4. Seek specialist advice if gout occurs in a person less than 25 years of age.
5. Stop allopurinol during an acute attack of gout.

Relevant literature

www.cks.nhs.uk/gout/management/quick_answers/scenario_acute_gout

http://arthritis.about.com/od/gout/a/foodstoeat.htm

Case 8 – Achilles tendinosis

Brief to the doctor

Mr GH is a 33 year old man who consults because of an Achilles tendon problem and would like a referral letter to a private physiotherapist.

Patient summary

Name	GH
Date of birth (Age)	33
Social and family history	Married Estate agent Marathon runner
Past medical history	Nil relevant
Current medication	Ibuprofen 400 mg prn

Tasks for the doctor

In this case, the tasks are to:
- clarify and assess the patient's symptoms
- negotiate an appropriate management plan

Brief to the patient – more about the patient

1. Profile:

- GH is a 33 year old estate agent
- married with 2 children aged 7 and 5 years
- he has run the London marathon for charity for the last 5 years and trains 6 days a week
- 4 months ago he started to notice a gradual onset of pain and stiffness in his left calf on waking and this was eased by a hot shower or by walking; this pain has become more severe and it is now interfering with his running

2. He is seeing the doctor today because:

- having researched the subject on the internet and in running magazines, he would like a letter of referral to a private physiotherapist he has located who specialises in sports injuries. He requires the letter in order to recoup the fees on his private health insurance.

3. Additional information:

- If the doctor asks specifically:
  - the onset of symptoms coincided with changing his running route to include hills, as he wanted to increase the workload and decrease the miles covered so that his training was less time-consuming
  - he has had the same running shoes for 7 months – he has always bought anti-pronation running shoes following an assessment in a specialist running footwear shop
- He believes GPs have no expertise in sports medicine and are not sympathetic to the demands of athletes; consequently:
  - he believes this consultation is a waste of time and he is annoyed that he has to see a doctor just to get a referral letter to someone he is paying to see
  - he is not prepared to take any medication or advice from the doctor
  - he is not prepared to be examined
- He is concerned that he will develop a chronic problem that will end his running days completely.

Approach to be taken

A. Data gathering, examination and clinical assessment skills

1. *Define the clinical problem: clarify why the patient has presented today*
   The doctor:
   - reads the patient information provided prior to the consultation
   - asks open questions to explore and clarify Mr GH's symptoms and what he has learned about the condition from his research on the internet and in magazines
   - empathises with his frustration at the restriction of his running schedule
   - asks closed questions to clarify details about possible predisposing factors that might require specific treatment or further referral
   - discovers Mr GH's belief that GPs have no expertise in sports injuries and are not sympathetic to athletes when they are injured
   - uses internal summaries: "*Can I just recap to make sure I have got things right?*"

2. *Performs an appropriate physical or mental examination*
   - In this case, an examination would normally be performed, but the patient refuses to be examined.
   - The need for an examination is explained in appropriate language –
     "*I would like to examine you in order to ensure that physiotherapy treatment is appropriate before I make a referral.*"

B. Clinical management skills

3. *Make an appropriate working diagnosis*
   - The doctor, based on the history, makes a working diagnosis of Achilles tendinopathy.

4. *Explain the problem to the patient using appropriate language*
   The doctor:
   - asks "*What do you know about this problem?*"
   - asks "*Does my explanation make sense? Is there anything else you would like to know?*"
   - explains why private insurers require referral letters

5. *Provide holistic care and use resources effectively*
   - The doctor understands socioeconomic/cultural background: "*It must be very frustrating not being able to run like you used to*"

6. *Prescribe appropriately*
   - The doctor agrees that a physiotherapy referral is appropriate in the first instance and that a physiotherapist with a special interest would be especially beneficial.

7. *Specify the conditions and interval for follow-up*
   - The doctor offers a follow-up appointment if Mr GH does not respond to physiotherapy.

C. Interpersonal skills: know and treat this patient

8. *Achieve rapport*
   The doctor:
   - listens attentively to Mr GH's concerns about his condition
   - explores and clarifies Mr GH's beliefs about GPs' competence in managing sports injuries, but is non-confrontational and non-judgemental
   - understands his request for referral to a specialist physiotherapist
   - shows empathy with Mr GH over his frustration at not being able to train normally and with having to see a doctor for a referral letter

9. *Give the patient the opportunity to be involved in significant management decisions*
   The doctor:
   - actively confirms the patient's understanding of the problem – "*Can I check what you have found out about your problem?*"
   - shares thoughts/involves patient – "*I think you're right to want to see a specialist physio as this problem can be difficult to treat*"

Debrief

Discuss how the doctor could, if needed, improve his performance. In particular, assess how the doctor:

- establishes rapport
- deals with Mr GH's beliefs about GPs' knowledge of sports injuries and sympathy with athletes
- deals with Mr GH's anger at having to consult in order to get a referral letter

Revising data gathering

What questions could the doctor ask to discover the patient's ideas, concerns, expectations and health beliefs?

- Ideas: *"You have done some research for yourself; what have you learned about treatments for your condition?"*
- Concerns: *"Are you worried about the long-term effects of your condition?"*
- Expectations: *"Would you like to ask me about treatments other than physiotherapy?"*
- Health beliefs: *"You don't seem to be very happy about having to see me today, is there a reason for that?"*

Test your theoretical knowledge

For each of the following statements, answer true (T) or false (F).

1. Some antibiotics have been linked with tendinopathies
2. Achilles tendinopathy usually has a good prognosis
3. When examined there is always an area of tenderness and thickening
4. In the acute phase, a 7–15 mm heel raise may relieve pain
5. Histopathologically, in tendinosis, there is neovessel development, collagen fibre disarray and an intense inflammatory response
6. Evidence-based treatments include all of the following: heel-drop (eccentric) exercises, GTN patches, sclerosing injections, and peritendinous corticosteroid injections.

Relevant literature

Alfredson H, Pietila T, Jonsson P, Lorentzon R. (1988) Heavy-load eccentric calf muscle training for the treatment of chronic Achilles tendinosis. *Am J Sports Med,* **26:** 360–366.

Alfredson H, Khan K, Cook J. (2006) An algorithm for managing Achilles tendinopathy: a primary care emphasis on treatment. *Physician Sports Med,* **34**

Case 9 – Heel pain

Brief to the doctor

Mr TP is a 28 year old man who presents with a painful left heel. He says that he saw your colleague, Dr Brown, 3 weeks ago and was told he would be referred to physiotherapy. When he phoned the local physiotherapy unit, he was informed that they hadn't received his referral. He still has heel pain.

Patient summary

Name   TP

Date of birth (Age)   28

Social and Family History Married, with a baby aged 8 weeks

Past medical history   Insurance medical for mortgage 2 years ago – nil of note

Acute medication   Diclofenac 50 mg thrice daily × 60 tablets

Consultation note by Dr Brown (three weeks ago):
'Actuary with gradual onset (4 weeks) L heel pain, worse medially. Started with morning pain and worse after activity. Now unable to finish rugby game over weekend because of 8/10 pain – walked off field. O/E: tender anterior to heel. Impression: typical plantar fasciitis. Plan: diclofenac × 60T and refer to physiotherapy.' (However, there is no referral letter attached to the consultation.)

Tasks for the doctor

In this case, the tasks are to:
- review what has happened since his previous consultation
- decide whether you need to re-examine
- clarify Mr TP's expectations of this consultation and if appropriate, try to meet them

Brief to the patient – more about the patient

1. Profile:

- Mr TP is a 28 year old actuary who works in the city centre
- he commutes to work by train; this is a busy service and occasionally he has to stand for 20 minutes before he can get a seat.
- married with 1 child, aged 8 weeks – she wakes at night and he has to help bottle-feed; he finds the night walking with baby painful
- Mr TP has never been ill before and is worried about his foot; he assumed he would make a quick recovery once he rested the foot for a couple of weeks

2. He is seeing the doctor today because:

- he called the physiotherapy unit to initiate an appointment and found out they hadn't received a referral letter – he wants to know what happened
- his foot still hurts despite rest and ice for 3 weeks – what should he do?
- he was informed by one of his rugby colleagues that an X-ray may be needed to see if he has a heel spur – should he have an X-ray?

3. Additional information:

- if the doctor does not offer him a suitable explanation or apology for what happened to his referral, he becomes increasingly irritated and overtly unhappy
- if the doctor offers him a private referral, he asks if the practice will pay for it as they inadvertently delayed his treatment
- if the doctor offers him a follow-up appointment in the surgery for a steroid injection, he asks for the risks and benefits and chooses not to have this done
- if the doctor gives him advice that will help him while he waits for his NHS physiotherapy appointment, he leaves feeling 'something has been done' and appears slightly appeased

Approach to be taken

A. Data gathering, examination and clinical assessment skills

1. *Define the clinical problem: clarify why the patient has presented today*
   The doctor:
   - reads the patient information provided prior to the consultation and is alerted by the absence of a referral letter
   - asks open questions to explore what Mr TP expects of today's consultation, thereby eliciting a history of the missing physiotherapy referral and on-going left heel pain
   - acknowledges both issues and empathises with his feelings of anxiety and frustration, for example, *"The absence of a referral letter both at the physiotherapy department and here in your notes does not look too promising, does it? I can see how you could be feeling worried about being let down. I don't know what has happened, but I promise you I will look into it and try to resolve this as best I can. Now, I haven't seen you before so I need to ask you some questions so that I can help you."*
   - asks closed questions to clarify details about the current symptoms and treatments tried
   - excludes red flags such as morning stiffness, back and buttock pain, and tenderness in ligament insertions in the extremities (symptoms of Reiter's disease or ankylosing spondylitis – a small minority of these patients present with plantar fasciitis); this set of questions could be signposted by saying, *"To rule out serious illness I need to ask you a few quick questions. Are your joints stiff in the morning; do you have pain in the…"*
   - explores the impact of the symptoms on his work and home life
   - discovers Mr TP's idea that plantar fasciitis should improve within 3 weeks, especially if the foot is rested and NSAIDs taken
   - discovers Mr TP's concern about having to wait even longer for an NHS physiotherapy appointment
   - discovers Mr TP's expectation of practical help in alleviating the pain and aiding recovery

2. *Performs an appropriate physical or mental examination*
   - In this case, because the history and examination findings of the previous consultation are so typical of plantar fasciitis, an examination is not required.
   - However, if examined, the patient is tender in front of the left heel.
   - The foot may have a high arch or may be flat (pes cavus or planus).
   - When walking, the medial arch (observed from behind) drops, creating a flat foot that rolls in (see www.sportsinjuryclinic.net/cybertherapist/front/foot/plantarfaciitis.htm).
   - Mr TP does not appear to be overweight.

B. Clinical management skills

3. *Make an appropriate working diagnosis*
   - The doctor, based on the typical history, makes a working diagnosis of plantar fasciitis.

4. *Explain the problem to the patient using appropriate language*
   The doctor:
   - having established that Mr TP knows about plantar fasciitis from his previous consultation, addresses his agenda
   - suggests that his idea that plantar fasciitis resolves quickly may be optimistic: studies show that most cases resolve by 6–12 months, but 5% of patients end up undergoing surgery for plantar fascia release when conservative measures fail (http://emedicine.medscape.com/article/86143-treatment)
   - negotiates a physiotherapy referral; offer to add in a paragraph explaining that the patient had consulted 3 weeks ago and the original referral is missing. Ask Mr TP if he could be available for short notice appointments if other patients cancel and indicate his availability and/or flexibility on the referral document.
   - address his expectation of practical advice: discuss footwear, orthotics, silicone heel pads, steroid injections, self massage by rolling the foot on a golf ball, stretching and strengthening exercises (www.aafp.org/afp/20010201/467.html); advise discontinuation of NSAIDs beyond 10 days
   - provides some information on the pros and cons of steroid injection – potential risks include rupture of the plantar fascia and fat pad atrophy
   - provides information on X-rays: plantar fasciitis produces heel spurs; heel spurs do not produce plantar fasciitis, hence, the spur, if present, should not be surgically removed; an X-ray may not add to the management

5. *Provide holistic care and use resources effectively*
   The doctor:
   - practises evidence-based medicine (http://emedicine.medscape.com/article/86143-treatment)
   - if Mr TP has a good basic understanding of plantar fasciitis, the doctor should build on this knowledge by discussing exercises (foot biomechanics) and self-help treatments

6. *Prescribe appropriately*
   The doctor:
   - checks the patient's understanding of NSAIDs, efficacy and side effects. The doctor suggests appropriate alternative analgesia.

7. *Specify the conditions and interval for follow-up*
   - The doctor offers a follow-up appointment, either to provide a steroid injection or to discuss any issues arising from the physiotherapy.

C. Interpersonal skills: know and treat this patient

8. *Achieve rapport*
   The doctor:
   - listens attentively to Mr TP's opening statements and acknowledges his feelings of fear, anxiety and frustration
   - deals with his anger at the 'lost' referral without placing undue blame on other members of staff
   - displays empathy with regard to the duration of illness and its adverse consequences
   - addresses the patient's specific concerns and expectations and encourages self-help

9. *Give the patient the opportunity to be involved in significant management decisions*
   - The doctor encourages autonomy and opinions – provides him with treatment options, discusses their risks and benefits and facilitates the patient's choice.

Debrief

Discuss how the doctor could, if needed, improve his performance. In particular, assess whether the doctor:

- was able to able to ask the appropriate 'red flag' questions?
- discussed prognosis? If so, was the language used simple and understandable?
- checked the patient's understanding? How did the doctor do this?
- established rapport and defused the patient's anger? If so, how?

If the consultation over-ran, did the doctor:

- re-take a history of the original presentation instead of focusing on what had happened in the interim?
- perform unnecessary examinations or take too long to examine?
- spend too much time placating the 'angry' patient and too little time addressing his need for on-going treatment?

Revising data gathering

What questions could the doctor ask to discover the patient's ideas, concerns, expectations and health beliefs?

- Ideas: *"How long, do you think, it takes for plantar fasciitis to get better?"*
- Concerns: *"The physiotherapy department has not received your referral. What do you suspect has happened?"*
- Expectations: *"You seem to have a good understanding of plantar fasciitis. What specific issues would you like me to address in today's consultation?"*
- Health beliefs: *"You mentioned getting an X-ray to look for heel spurs. Let's discuss this further"*

Test your theoretical knowledge

For each of the following statements, answer true (T) or false (F).

Regarding plantar fasciitis:

1. The pain is usually caused by collagen deposition at the origin of the plantar fascia at the lateral tubercle of the calcaneus.
2. The worst pain occurs with the first few steps in the morning.
3. Patients often notice pain at the end of activity that lessens or resolves as they rest.
4. Flat feet increases the risk for developing plantar fasciitis while high arches are protective.
5. The pain may be exacerbated by passive dorsiflexion of the toes.
6. The pain may be exacerbated by having the patient stand on the tips of the toes.
7. With age, running shoes retain their shock absorption; getting a new pair of shoes is likely to stretch the arch and increase the pain.
8. Some studies suggest that arch taping and orthotics may be better than NSAIDs or cortisone injection.

Relevant literature

www.aafp.org/afp/20010201/467.html

Case 10 – Acne

Brief to the doctor

Mr GH is a 24 year old man who consults because he has acne affecting his face and back.

Patient summary

Name	GH
Date of birth (Age)	24
Social and family history	Single Labourer
Past medical history	GP consultations: 14 months ago – "*Acne – face and shoulders. Pustules > comedones. For oxytetracycline 250 mg 2 bd 3/12*"
	11 months ago – "*Acne review. No improvement after 3/12 oxytet, add benzoyl peroxide gel. Warned re irritation and bleaching.*"
Current medication	None No recorded allergies
Investigations	None

Tasks for the doctor

In this case, the tasks are to:
- review previous medication and try to identify why he has not responded
- identify Mr GH's concerns about his acne and offer support
- prescribe appropriately

Brief to the patient – more about the patient

1. Profile:

- Mr GH is a 24 year old single man
- he works as a labourer on a building site

2. He is seeing the doctor today because:

- he has had acne (spots and blackheads) on his face and back for just over a year and is concerned about the cosmetic appearance
- he saw a GP last year and was given a 3 month course of oxytetracycline without any real benefit; benzoyl peroxide was then added, but again this did not help; he did not bother going back
- he is training to take part in a body building competition – he feels he will not score well in the competition if he is 'spotty'

3. Additional information:

- He was not troubled by acne as a teenager; his voice broke age 11 and he started shaving at 14, by which age he was 6' 1" tall.
- If the doctor asks specifically:
  - he does not come into contact with any chemicals at work
  - for the last 18 months he has been using protein supplements which he buys at the gym
  - most of the other body builders at the gym use steroid tablets and injections
  - he follows a high protein high carbohydrate diet
  - his girlfriend recently split up with him after 4 years together because she was fed up with him always being at the gym and said that he had been become moody and snappy
  - he is not sleeping well; he has no depressive symptoms
- He believes he can train and do well 'naturally'; he refuses to use steroids because he has heard they have long-term effects that are irreversible.
- His trainer has pressured him on several occasions to use steroids. Taking the protein supplements was a compromise that Mr GH complied with to get his trainer 'off his back'.
- He is not aware that some supplements have been reported to contain traces of androgenic-anabolic steroids.
- If the doctor performs an examination:

System	Findings
General	Very well built fit young man No jaundice. No gynaecomastia. Normal body hair
Skin	Comedones and pustules on face, shoulders and back. No scarring or cysts.
Cardiovascular	BP 134/88 (use large cuff)
Abdomen	No enlarged liver No evidence of testicular atrophy

Approach to be taken

A. Data gathering, examination and clinical assessment skills

1. *Define the clinical problem: clarify why the patient has presented today*
   The doctor:
   - reads the patient information provided prior to the consultation
   - asks open questions to explore:
     - whether Mr GH had acne in the past and how it was treated
     - why he is concerned about his acne at this time
     - whether the acne is having any psychosocial effects on him– *"How is this affecting you?"*
     - whether Mr GH has considered that the protein supplements might contain traces of androgenic-anabolic steroids and that this might be the cause of his acne – *"Some sports supplements have been found to contain traces of anabolic steroids and other substances – have you ever wondered about this?"*
   - asks closed questions to:
     - exclude other causes of rashes – *"As a builder, do you come into contact with any irritant chemicals that might cause this?"*
     - be sure that he is not knowingly using androgenic-anabolic steroids or other agents – *"I am sorry, but I have to ask this question because it will affect how we treat your problem. Are you taking any supplements or other substances to enhance your performance or physique?"*
     - assess if he has experienced other possible unwanted effects of androgenic-anabolic steroids – psychological
   - empathises with Mr GH about:
     - the cosmetic effects and having acne occur for the first time at his age rather than in his teens: *"It must be a bit of a shock starting to get acne as an adult rather than as a teenager. How are you coping with that?"*
     - his feelings about androgenic-anabolic steroid use: *"You have heard that anabolic steroids have some serious side-effects, would you like to discuss this?"*

2. *Performs an appropriate physical or mental examination*
   - In this case, a targeted examination is required. A minimally acceptable examination would be, with the patient's shirt removed:
     - examination of the acne to confirm the diagnosis and assess severity
     - a quick visual check to exclude gynaecomastia, loss of body hair, and liver disease stigmata
   - If time permits, a BP check could be done, although this could be deferred to a follow up appointment, given that there are no other signs of anabolic steroid use.
   - The need for an examination should be explained in appropriate language.

B. Clinical management skills

3. *Make an appropriate working diagnosis*
   - The doctor integrates information and makes a working diagnosis of acne probably secondary to androgenic-anabolic steroid use.
   - This is a clinically sound hypothesis with an appropriate use of probability.

4. *Explain the problem to the patient using appropriate language*
   The doctor:
   - having established Mr GH's feelings about drugs, sensitively explains that some protein supplements have been reported to contain androgenic-anabolic steroids – *"If I were to say to you that some supplements have been reported to contain anabolic steroids, how would you feel?"*
   - explains that acne is a reported unwanted effect of androgenic-anabolic steroids
   - provides information on androgenic-anabolic steroids to include unwanted effects
   - advises Mr GH that the unwanted effects are largely reversible if androgenic-anabolic steroid use is stopped
   - uses chunking and checking of information to evaluate Gary's understanding: *"I have given you a lot of unexpected information, before I examine you, can I just check that I have explained things clearly?"*

5. *Provide holistic care and use resources effectively*
   The doctor:
   - builds on Mr GH's health beliefs to identify management options – *"You've told me that you are against drugs, would you be happy to stop using the supplements and see if the problem goes away?"*
   - understands socioeconomic/cultural background – *"Are you concerned that stopping the supplements might affect your chances in the competition?"*
   - discusses with Mr GH whether to perform blood tests to look for biochemical effects of androgenic-anabolic steroids – *"It is possible that you may have been taking a supplement that contains steroids and that this is the cause of your acne. We have talked about some of the side effects of these. Would you like to have a blood test to check whether there are any signs of other side effects?"*

6. *Prescribe appropriately*
   - The doctor agrees an appropriate management plan with the patient to include:
     - that Mr GH should stop taking the protein supplements and be reviewed in a month to see if his acne had improved
     - having blood tests – FBC, U&Es, LFTs, fasting glucose and fasting lipids

7. *Specify the conditions and interval for follow-up*
   - The doctor arranged a follow-up appointment to monitor progress of the acne and review the blood test results.

C. Interpersonal skills: know and treat this patient

8. *Achieve rapport*
   The doctor:
   - listens attentively
   - follows up verbal and non-verbal cues – *"You mentioned body-building, I know that some body builders use special supplements to improve their performance..."*
   - sensitively explores and clarifies Mr GH's supplement use and his feelings about androgenic-anabolic steroids
   - places the problem in a psychosocial context – how it affects patient/relationships: *"You mentioned that your girlfriend said you were moody and snappy, was this just with her?"*
   - is non-judgemental about Mr GH's use of protein supplements
   - empathises with Mr GH about getting acne in adult life

9. *Give the patient the opportunity to be involved in significant management decisions*
   The doctor:
   - actively confirms patient's understanding of the problem – *"Is there anything else you would like to ask?"*
   - shares thoughts with the patient that the protein supplements may be causing the acne
   - encourages autonomy by building on Mr GH's ideas and concerns about taking anabolic steroids to agree a management plan

Debrief

Discuss how the doctor could, if needed, improve his performance. In particular, assess how the doctor:

- established rapport and identified Mr GH's beliefs about androgenic-anabolic steroid use
- raised the possibility of the supplements containing androgenic-anabolic steroids and that this might be the cause of his acne

Revising data gathering

What questions could the doctor ask to discover the patient's ideas, concerns, expectations and health beliefs?

- Ideas: *"I understand that you are surprised that you have started getting acne at your age, do you have any ideas why this has happened now?"*
- Concerns: *"Are you concerned that you might have other side effects of anabolic steroids?"*
- Expectations: *"Would you like to have some blood tests to see if there are any signs of other steroid side effects?"*
- Health beliefs: *"You said that you are worried about the long-term effects of androgenic-anabolic steroids, would you like to discuss this?"*

Test your theoretical knowledge

For each of the following statements, answer true (T) or false (F).

1. The requirements for protein and calories appear to increase when training with the aid of anabolic-androgenic steroids
2. Anabolic-androgenic steroids remain detectable for several weeks whether taken orally or by injection
3. Drugs on the World Anti-Doping Agency 'banned list' include all beta 2 agonists, tamoxifen, and thiazide diuretics
4. Anabolic-androgenic steroids may induce hyperinsulinism
5. Regimens for using anabolic-androgenic steroids include stacking, pyramids, and tapering
6. Before more effective drugs were available, anabolic-androgenic steroids had been used to treat depression and other mental health disorders

Relevant literature

Bahrke MS, Yesalis CE. (2002) *Performance-Enhancing Substances in Sport and Exercise.* Human Kinetics, Champaign Illinois.

World Anti-Doping Agency (WADA) website: www.wada-ama.org

WADA Athlete guide:
www.wada-ama.org/rtecontent/document/WADA_Athlete-Guide_ENG.pdf

Case 11 – Post-partum problems

Brief to the doctor

Mrs PH is a 32 year old woman who is added to the end of your clinic as a telephone consultation. You call her back on the number supplied. Mrs PH saw the practice nurse 4 days ago for blood tests.

Patient summary

Name	PH
Date of birth (Age)	34
Social and Family History	Married with two children Her son was born 10 days ago
Past medical history	Heartburn during pregnancy
Current medication	Gaviscon as required

Consultation note by practice nurse (four days ago):
'Discharged from labour ward but advised to have FBC taken as loss of 850 ml blood. Is feeling light-headed but not SOB. Blood taken from L cubital fossa using aseptic technique. Patient advised to call surgery for results in 3–5 days.'

Blood tests	Tests were done four days ago
Hb	10.5 g/dl (12–15)
MCV	97 (83–105)
White cell count	6.67 (4–11)
Differential count	no abnormalities
Platelet count	285 (150–400)

Tasks for the doctor

In this case, the tasks are to:
- clarify, with attention to auditory cues, Mrs PH's reason(s) for calling
- take a detailed history
- actively confirm that the patient understands the treatment plan

Brief to the patient – more about the patient

1. Profile:

- Mrs PH is a 34 year old woman who is currently on maternity leave; her baby boy was born 10 days ago
- she is married and has an older daughter, aged 6
- Mrs PH wants the results of her blood tests; she was also advised by the health visitor to tell you about the 'clot' she has passed

2. She is calling the doctor today because:

- she would like to know the results of her recent blood tests and whether treatment is needed
- the health visitor advised her to tell the GP about the clot she passed: two days ago, she passed one small clot vaginally – it was the size of a 50 pence coin; the clot did not seem to contain any tissue and there have not been other clots or smelly discharge or abdominal pain
- when asked about the birth, she tells you that her waters broke at 2 pm, her labour progressed quickly, her baby was born by NVD at 10 pm, but she was then taken to theatre for a manual removal of placenta, hence the 850 ml loss of blood; she cannot remember if the she was given antibiotics intravenously at the time of the procedure and she was not given antibiotic tablets after the manual removal
- she feels well in herself and has not had fever or rigors
- her main concern is that treatments may interfere with her breastfeeding; she has had a few problems with breastfeeding, which is why she is seeing the health visitor for advice – she wants to breastfeed and would prefer to avoid formula milk if at all possible; she is wary of antibiotics, particularly if antibiotics pass into breast milk and give the baby diarrhoea, resulting in further weight loss
- she expects advice: what should she do about her blood results and her bleeding?

3. Additional information:

- if the doctor discusses an iron-rich diet, she says that she eats meat, bran, baked beans, etc. and has no problem avoiding tea and coffee with meals
- if the doctor suggests iron tablets, she says she has not had problems with iron tablets in the past – she expects the doctor to make arrangements for the prescription
- if you suggest a wait and see policy, she expects to be told when to seek your advice again
- if you suggest that she comes in to see a GP, she wants to know if she needs to attend today as arranging childcare for her 6 year old may be difficult

Approach to be taken

A. Data gathering, examination and clinical assessment skills

1. *Define the clinical problem: clarify why the patient has telephoned today*
   The doctor:
   - reads the patient information provided prior to the consultation and notes that Mrs HP lost 850 ml of blood during birth and now has an Hb of 10.6 g/dl
   - telephones Mrs HP on the number provided; he introduces himself and establishes the identity of the patient – if someone else answers, he asks to speak to the patient because a first-hand history is usually more reliable
   - clarifies the nature of the problem and understands exactly what the patient is requesting today; one approach is *"I see from your notes you recently gave birth. Congratulations! I also see that you had some blood tests done a few days ago. What can I do for you today?"*
   - asks open questions to explore the two issues raised by the patient, such as *"How are you feeling now?"* or *"Tell me more about the clots"*
   - asks closed questions to clarify details about the post-partum bleeding: fever, rigors, feeling unwell, racing pulse, risk factors for endometritis, such as a manual removal of placenta; by asking about current infection, the doctor systematically excludes red flags signalling the need for review or referral
   - empathises with her difficulties in breastfeeding and elicits her concerns regarding treatments that may interfere with breastfeeding
   - elicits her expectations for advice regarding her two issues, namely anaemia and post-partum bleeding

2. *Performs an appropriate physical or mental examination*
   - In this case, an examination is not required. The difficulty with telephone triage is the ability to make management decisions in the absence of visual cues.

B. Clinical management skills

3. *Make an appropriate working diagnosis*
   - The doctor, based on the history, makes a working diagnosis of (1) anaemia due to blood loss at delivery, and (2) the possibility of secondary post-partum haemorrhage (PPH) due to endometrial infection.

4. *Explain the problem to the patient using appropriate language*
   The doctor:
   - addresses Mrs PH's agenda: what does Mrs PH know about dietary treatments for anaemia / iron tablets / fluids that reduce iron absorption? The doctor may explain why he is concerned about the PV bleeding – that it could be a warning sign of 'hidden infection in the womb'

- gives the information about PPH in digestable chunks: a severe case of PPH would have more bleeding or purulent lochia, the patient would feel unwell (like flu), have a racing pulse, feel flushed and feverish, with sweating that wets the clothes; the patient's understanding is checked at each step
- addresses Mrs PH's concerns: an iron-rich diet, with or without iron tablets, is unlikely to interfere with breastfeeding; further assessment of the vaginal bleed may be needed in the form of a pelvic examination – she may not want her 6 year old daughter present during this examination (or the curtains could be drawn around the bed for privacy) – the assessment could take place within the next few days, at her convenience; however, if symptoms of severe infection develop, she needs to see a doctor urgently
- 'prescribes' an iron-rich diet and negotiates prescription of iron tablets according to Mrs PH's preferences

5. *Provide holistic care and use resources effectively*
   The doctor:
   - manages both problems (anaemia and PV bleeding) in accordance with national or local guidelines
   - checks that there is agreement and understanding with what is proposed
   - does not waste time addressing the breastfeeding issue if Mrs CC is happy with the advice she has received from the health visitor – the time is better spent addressing her concerns about anaemia and PV bleeding

6. *Prescribe appropriately*
   The doctor:
   - is aware of national and local guidelines – www.nice.org.uk/nicemedia/pdf/CG037fullguideline.pdf (pages 113–125) and www.bsg.org.uk/pdf_word_docs/iron_def.pdf
   - if prescribing, discusses how iron tablets are taken and the commonly experienced side effects

7. *Specify the conditions and interval for follow-up*
   The doctor:
   - arranges the follow-up appointment for the pelvic examination
   - outlines the red flag symptoms; if these symptoms develop, Mrs PH should seek urgent care (i.e safety-nets)
   - summarises, for example, with *"Just to recap, we've agreed that you will eat more red meat and cornflakes and avoid tea and coffee with meals. Your husband will collect the prescription for iron tablets and you will take one tablet daily with orange juice. You will keep an eye on your vaginal bleeding. If it is settling you will see me for an examination at your convenience in the next few days. If you develop a temperature, more bleeding, or start to feel unwell, you will ring back and I will see you as an emergency appointment. Are you happy with these arrangements?"*

C. Interpersonal skills: know and treat this patient

8. *Achieve rapport*
   The doctor:
   - listens attentively to Mrs PH's request for advice, does not interrupt unnecessarily, and maintains the flow of conversation
   - questions in a systematic manner, taking care to deal with one issue at a time
   - is sensitive in his queries and ensures that the conversation does not sound like an interrogation
   - understands the patient's request for advice and refrains from making comments such as *"I don't know why the health visitor didn't sort this out herself!"*
   - displays empathy to her predicament – *"I can understand why you'd prefer to avoid any tablets that interfere with the breastfeeding routine you've worked so hard to establish. Let me reassure you that iron tablets will not affect the feeding."*
   - is alert to the possibility of PPH in someone who has had a manual removal of the placenta; however, he does not alarm the patient unduly

9. *Give the patient the opportunity to be involved in significant management decisions*
   - The doctor encourages autonomy and opinions – provides the patient with information on diet and iron tablets and allows her to choose her own treatment; provides sufficient information on why a pelvic examination may be needed and Mrs PH is able to make an appointment that fits in with her childcare

Debrief

Discuss how the doctor could, if needed, improve his performance. In particular, assess whether the doctor:
- established rapport on the telephone? If so, how?
- established the patient's reasons for calling? If so, how?
- dealt with Mrs PH's specific concerns in a systematic manner? If so, how?
- discussed the red flags for PPH in a non-alarmist manner?
- summarised and checked understanding?

If the consultation over-ran, did the doctor:
- interrupt unnecessarily?
- get side-tracked by other issues, such as breastfeeding, that Mrs PH was happy to leave to the health visitor?
- repeat some explanations and reassurances?

Revising data gathering

What questions could the doctor ask to discover the patient's ideas, concerns, expectations and health beliefs?
- Ideas: *"Do you have any ideas on how anaemia (low blood counts) is treated?"*
- Concerns: *"Regarding the clot, did you have any worries about what might be happening?"*
- Expectations: *"It seems to me that you want a treatment that does not interfere with your breastfeeding. Do I understand you correctly?"*
- Health beliefs: *"You sound as if you suspect that something is not quite right if you pass a clot a week after delivering. Let's talk about this for a moment."*

Test your theoretical knowledge

For each of the following statements, answer true (T) or false (F).
1. The WHO classifies anaemia in non-pregnant women, over 15 years, as an Hb < 12 g/dl.
2. The WHO classifies anaemia in pregnant women, as an Hb < 10 g/dl.
3. If iron deficiency anaemia co-exists with a B12 or folate deficiency, the red cell distribution width (RDW) is decreased.
4. Continue oral iron therapy (ferrous sulphate 200 mg twice daily) for three months after the iron deficiency has been corrected to replenish stores.
5. Teenage girls and women under 50 years should have 14.8 mg of iron a day.
6. A 125 g can of sardines in tomato sauce contains less iron than two slices of lean roast beef.
7. A 30 g bowl of branflakes and a 30 g bowl cornflakes contain equivalent amounts of iron.

Relevant literature

www.weightlossresources.co.uk/diet/healthy_diet/iron_rich_food.htm

www.bsg.org.uk/pdf_word_docs/iron_def.pdf

Case 12 – Relative with bowel cancer

Brief to the doctor

Mr KL is a 20 year old man who presents in a routine surgery. He has registered as a temporary resident as he is in his first year at university. He has come home because his father has recently had surgery for bowel cancer at the age of 44 years. He has asked to talk about genetic screening for bowel cancer with a doctor. Mr KL saw one of your partners last year, just before he left to go to university, when he had noticed some blood on the toilet paper for a few days, but he was told not to worry.

Patient summary

Name	KL
Date of birth (Age)	20
Social and family history	Student Father diagnosed with cancer of the bowel 2 months ago
Past medical history	GP consultation: 1 year ago – *"c/o fresh blood on toilet paper when he wipes – 4 days, none in pan. Stool normal but has been straining a bit. Well in self. No pain. Prob pile. Reassured, told to return if continues."*
Current medication	None
Investigations	None

Tasks for the doctor

In this case, the tasks are to:
- confirm details of his father's diagnosis and any advice given for relatives by the hospital consultant, while respecting KL's father's right to confidentiality; as a result discuss whether Mr KL should be referred for genetic advice and screening
- explore Mr KL's concerns about his rectal bleeding last year
- discuss symptoms and factors linked with bowel cancer, including genetics; discuss any lifestyle changes Mr KL may like to make

Brief to the patient – more about the patient

1. Profile:

- Mr KL is a 20 year old Sports Science student
- he lives in a hall of residence but tends not to eat there as he often goes to the gym in the evenings and so has takeaways or Pot Noodles in the evenings
- he saw one of the GPs in this practice a year ago because he had had some rectal bleeding and was told he probably had a pile and need not worry. He has had a couple of episodes of fresh blood on the paper since then. His health is excellent – he feels well and has not lost weight.
- his father had rectal bleeding 6 months ago and saw the same partner KL saw last year and the father was also told he probably had piles and not to worry – he then saw another partner and was referred to the hospital 2 months ago. Mr KL's father has told him that he had a 'Stage 2' tumour. His father has had a right hemicolectomy and is going to have chemotherapy.
- Mr KL is angry that his father was not referred earlier by your partner and concerned that he had the same symptoms and was also 'fobbed off' without an examination
- Mr KL believes that lifestyle has a major effect on health and is very open to health promotion advice – he feels guilty that he has neglected his own diet
- he has not looked up bowel cancer on the internet yet as he has not had time, but intends to do so

2. He is seeing the doctor today because:

- he wants information on the genetics of bowel cancer and advice on whether he should have screening; he would like to discuss what screening tests are possible and their accuracy
- he would like to be reassured about his own rectal bleeding and would like to be told exactly what the cause is – he feels he should be examined and referred to a specialist
- he wants advice on what preventive measures he can take

3. Addditional information:

- If the doctor examines him:

System	Findings
General	Well. No evidence of weight loss No pallor
Abdomen	Soft. No tenderness No masses or organomegaly
Rectal examination	Perianal skin – NAD. No external piles/skin tags Empty rectum. No masses felt. No blood on glove

Approach to be taken

A. Data gathering, examination and clinical assessment skills

1. Define the clinical problem: clarify why the patient has presented today
The doctor:

- reads the patient information provided prior to the consultation
- asks open questions to clarify details of:
  - Mr KL's father's condition – *"I haven't got your father's records, tell me about him."*
  - Mr KL's concerns for himself – *"You seem concerned that you have the same symptoms as your father?"*
  - Mr KL's request for information on genetic screening – *"What do you know about screening for bowel cancer?"*
  - Mr KL's knowledge about causes of the condition
- asks closed questions to clarify:
  - details of Mr KL's own symptoms to exclude red flag symptoms signalling the need for review or referral
  - what advice, if any, the hospital has given about screening the rest of the family
- uses internal summaries – *"Can I just check I've got things right…"*

2. Performs an appropriate physical or mental examination

- In this case, an examination is required to address the patient's concerns.
- The examination should be explained in appropriate language – *"I need to examine your abdomen and then do an internal examination with a finger."*
- A targeted examination should be performed – abdomen and RE.

B. Clinical management skills

3. Make an appropriate working diagnosis

- The doctor, based on the history and examination, makes a working diagnosis of haemorrhoidal bleeding.
- This is a clinically sound hypothesis and makes an appropriate use of probability.

4. Explain the problem to the patient using appropriate language
The doctor:

- explains the likely cause of Mr KL's symptoms
- addresses Mr KL's agenda:
  - that he should be referred to ensure he does not have cancer
  - discusses factors associated with bowel cancer pertinent to him including diet and genetics: *"What do you know about causes of bowel cancer?"*
  - discusses screening for bowel cancer: *"Do you know much about screening for bowel cancer?"*

- addresses Mr KL's concerns about the management of his father in a non-judgemental way and respecting his father's confidentiality

5. *Provide holistic care and use resources effectively*
The doctor:
- practises evidence-based medicine using national guidelines – NICE (2005) *Referral guidelines for suspected cancer* (CG27 – www.nice.org.uk/Guidance/CG27)
- uses Mr KL's health beliefs to reinforce advice about preventive measures he could take – *"You seem to be keen on preventing cancers, would you like to discuss things you might be able to do to decrease your risks?"*
- respects his father's right to confidentiality – *"I am afraid I can't discuss details of your father's case without his permission. Can I suggest you discuss your concerns with your family to see if they share your feelings?"*
- advises Mr KL about the complaints procedure – *"Would you like me to give you details of how to make a complaint, if you and your family decide to do so?"*

6. *Prescribe appropriately*
The doctor:
- chooses to advise Mr KL about diet rather than provide local treatments (haemorrhoid creams) for the management of his symptoms
- writes to Mr KL's father's consultant to ask if Mr KL should also be referred for screening as his father had developed bowel cancer before the age of 45, with a copy to Mr KL's GP at university for information

7. *Specify the conditions and interval for follow-up*
The doctor:
- offers a follow-up appointment to discuss any issues arising from Mr KL's own symptoms, lifestyle change and his father's condition
- checks understanding: *"Just to check that I have explained things clearly, can you tell me what we have agreed to do today?"*

C. Interpersonal skills: know and treat this patient

8. *Achieve rapport*
The doctor:
- listens attentively to Mr KL's concerns about:
  - his father's condition and perceived delayed referral
  - his own symptoms and his risk of developing bowel cancer in the future
- explores and clarifies Mr KL's health beliefs and concerns – that lifestyle contributes to maintaining health
- understands his request for information on screening and genetic counselling
- is non-judgemental about the patient's ideas on his father's management, but expresses sympathy with Mr KL's feelings and upset

9. *Give the patient the opportunity to be involved in significant management decisions*
   The doctor:
   - actively confirms the patient's understanding of the problem: *"Does my explanation of the likely cause of your symptoms sound reasonable to you?"*
   - balances plans – doctor/patient centred as appropriate – *"I don't think I need to refer you about your bleeding at the moment, but agree it would be sensible to check with the hospital whether your father had one of the sorts of cancer that might have a genetic component, in which case you will need to be referred"*

Debrief

Discuss how the doctor could, if needed, improve his performance. In particular, assess how the doctor:

- obtained information about Mr KL's father's cancer to enable him to answer Mr KL's questions. Did he get all the necessary information from Mr KL or could he have consulted the father's medical records? What are the issues relating to discussing his father's records with Mr KL?
- dealt with Mr KL's rectal bleeding symptoms. Was an examination appropriate or necessary? Should a chaperone be offered?
- dealt with Mr KL's anger over his partner's advice to both Mr KL and his father
- gained Mr KL's trust

Revising data gathering

What questions could the doctor ask to discover the patient's ideas, concerns, expectations and health beliefs?

- Ideas: *"You seem to be angry about the advice the other doctor gave you and your father; would you like to discuss that?"*
- Concerns: *"Are you worried that you might develop bowel cancer at some time in the future?"*
- Expectations: *"You said you were unhappy that my partner didn't examine you last year; would you prefer to be examined today?"* and *"I understand your anxiety about your own symptoms and why you would like an exact diagnosis, how were you hoping I would help with those today?"*
- Health beliefs: *"Being fit and healthy is important to you; would you like to discuss things you can do that might decrease your chances of developing bowel cancer?"*

Once the doctor has gathered sufficient information, how could he summarise the problem for the patient?

- *"We have discussed a lot of things today, can I just summarise them to make sure I have covered all the things you wanted and that we have agreed on what to do about them all?"*
- *"Are you happy with what we have covered or do you have any questions or concerns?"*

Test your theoretical knowledge

For each of the following statements, answer true (T) or false (F).

1. Bowel cancer is the second commonest cause of cancer-related deaths in Western countries
2. Dietary factors play a minimal role in developing bowel cancer
3. Trials have shown that aspirin 300 mg daily reduces the risk of bowel cancer by 20%

4. The commonest inherited form of bowel cancer is non-polyposis colon cancer (HNPCC or Lynch Syndrome)
5. Faecal occult blood (FOB) screening has a sensitivity of 90% for bowel cancers
6. Anyone over 55 with rectal bleeding, or anyone with a combination of rectal bleeding and altered bowel habit, should be seen at a hospital within 2 weeks of referral by their GP

Relevant literature

Jones R, Latinovic R, Charlton J, Gulliford MC. (2007) Alarm symptoms in early diagnosis of cancer in primary care: cohort study using General Practice Research Database. *BMJ,* **334:** 1040–1044.

Department of Health (2000) *Referral guidelines for suspected cancer.*

NICE (2005) *Referral guidelines for suspected cancer,* CG27: www.nice.org.uk/Guidance/CG27

Case 13 – Food poisoning

Brief to the doctor

Mr EJ is a 32 year old man who consulted your colleague, Dr Brown 5 days ago. The microbiology laboratory telephoned the practice nurse this morning to relay the results of Mr EJ's stool sample: campylobacter was isolated. The nurse added Mr EJ to your appointment list for you to telephone him with the results.

Patient summary

Name	EJ
Date of birth (Age)	32
Social and Family History	Unmarried; works as an airline steward
Past medical history	Low back pain 6 months ago Poor sleep pattern 2 years ago
Medication	None

Dr Brown's consultation (5 days ago)
'Diarrhoea symptoms: frequent, loose motions. Fresh blood from piles and no mucus. Passing watery stool every 1–2 hours. Crampy, abdominal pain – using NSAIDs and paracetamol. Recent travel to Jordan and Germany; stayed in hotels. Ate egg sandwich at Frankfurt airport. Had salmonella age 17. O/E: hydrated, slightly dry lips. Generalised abdominal tenderness. No guarding. T 37.3°C. Plan: get stool samples × 2.Use Imodium only if diarrhoea is interrupting sleep. Not due back at work for a few days.'

Tasks for the doctor

In this case, the tasks are to:
- contact Mr EJ with his results
- review his symptoms
- provide appropriate occupational advice

Brief to the patient – more about the patient

1. Profile:

- Mr EJ is a 32 year old man who works as a steward for a budget airline
- he is unmarried and lives alone; he has had several relationships with partners of the same sex. His last HIV test at the GUM clinic 3 months ago, after the break-up of his most recent relationship, was negative. He has used condoms since.
- Mr EJ feels ill and is worried about the abdominal cramp he is experiencing with this bout of food poisoning.

2. When the surgery contacts him, he updates them on his illness:

- the diarrhoea has improved but he does not feel completely well
- he passes two to three loose, not watery, stools daily and is now able to sleep through the night; he did not use any tablets to reduce stool frequency – he drank fluids to rehydrate and now tolerates bland food. He does not have nausea or vomiting.
- he still experiences generalised stomach cramp, unrelated to meals, but the cramp is not as severe (3/10) nor does it last as long (10 minutes) compared to 5 days ago
- he has been recuperating at home. However, he is due to fly to Spain on the early flight tomorrow and thinks he feels well enough to undertake the short-haul. He works several flights for the next 3 days after which he meets with friends in Spain where a party is planned.
- he is shocked to hear about the positive campylobacter result; he expected the cultures to be negative, and he wants to know if further treatment is needed
- he expects to return to work tomorrow – is this OK? As a steward, one of his duties is to sell packaged food and beverages on flights.
- does he need to inform work about his results?
- with regard to the party, is he OK to drink alcohol?
- Mr EJ is a chatty man and one of the difficulties in this case is to remain focused on the relevant medical issues

3. Additional information:

- if the doctor does not prescribe antibiotics, he wants to know if there could be complications later on?
- should he give a stool sample at a later date to check for eradication?
- if the doctor prescribes antibiotics, he wants to know if he can return to work within 24 hours – presumably he won't be infectious then?
- this is his 2nd bowel infection – is there something predisposing him to bowel infections? Is there anything he can do to prevent getting infections?

Approach to be taken

A. Data gathering, examination and clinical assessment skills

1. *Define the clinical problem: inform the patient of the results and clarify the issues a positive result has for him*
   The doctor:
   - reads the patient notes provided prior to the telephone consultation and thinks about what information he needs to obtain from Mr EJ
   - telephones Mr EJ on the number provided and introduces himself; he establishes the identity of the caller / patient and speaks to the patient directly
   - signposts or structures the consultations, for example, says *"Mr EJ, I have the results of your stool sample. Before we discuss these, I'd like to ask you some questions."*
   - asks open questions to explore how Mr EJ is feeling at the moment and, if there has been an improvement, what has improved and what helped him to feel better
   - asks closed questions to clarify details about fever, pain, diarrhoea (frequency, consistency, presence of blood or mucus) since he was last seen
   - asks about red flag symptoms (which may signal the need for antibiotics), namely feeling very unwell, having a high temperature, passing more than eight stools per day, being ill for longer than 1 week or being immunocompromised
   - empathises with the pain and disruption the diarrhoea has caused to Mr EJ's usual routine; clarifies the impact the illness has had on his family and work. The doctor is alert to the fact that Mr EJ is a food handler.
   - discovers Mr EJ's idea that his illness is a mild, self-limiting case of food poisoning, his expectation of returning to work as an airline steward tomorrow, and his concern about whether work should be informed about a positive campylobacter result

2. *Performs an appropriate physical or mental examination*
   - In this case, an examination is not required.

B. Clinical management skills

3. *Make an appropriate working diagnosis*
   - The doctor, based on the history, makes a working diagnosis of improving campylobacter diarrhoea. In the absence of red flag symptoms, antibiotics are not indicated. However, this needs to be balanced against his status as a food handler who, if not given antibiotics, may continue to shed organisms in the stool for up to 4 weeks. Infection usually occurs via infected food or

water; person-to-person transmission via the faeco-oral route is rare. In addition, Mr EJ handles packaged food so the risk of transmission is further reduced.

4. *Explain the problem to the patient using appropriate language*
   The doctor:
   - having established that Mr EJ is improving, informs him of his microbiology results
   - provides him with information about the natural history of campylobacter gastroenteritis and possible treatments: rehydration (200 ml after each loose stool), antibiotics in severe cases (erythromycin or ciprofloxacin), avoid antimotility drugs, and probiotics may help to reduce the duration of diarrhoea by 1 day
   - provides some occupational advice: all workers, including food handlers, are advised to return to work 48 hours after the last episode of diarrhoea
   - addresses Mr EJ's specific questions about possible complications (15% develop irritable bowel syndrome post-infection)

5. *Provide holistic care and use resources effectively*
   The doctor:
   - practises evidence-based medicine that is informed by national or local guidelines
   - informs Mr EJ about camplylobacter being a notifiable disease (search for "notifiable diseases" on www.hpa.org.uk)
   - if Mr EJ does not raise the issue of a sick note, the doctor (time permitting) may wish to inform him that notes are issued for sickness absences lasting more than 6 days
   - some companies offer flexible working patterns and if the patient is unable to attend work (e.g. with diarrhoea), then some work, especially if computer or internet based, can be done from home; patients are encouraged to liaise directly with their occupational health or human resources departments

6. *Prescribe appropriately*
   - The doctor is aware of national and local guidelines when making a decision on prescribing (http://cks.library.nhs.uk/mobiledevices/ckscontent.aspx?rawurl=gastroenteritis)

7. *Specify the conditions and interval for follow-up*
   The doctor:
   - discusses the 'red flag' symptoms and advises the patient to consult if these develop
   - if sick certification advice is provided, the advice is in line with national guidance (www.hpa.org.uk/cdph/issues/CDPHvol7/No4/guidelines2_4_04.pdf – see page 368)

C. Interpersonal skills: know and treat this patient

8. *Achieve rapport*
   The doctor:
   - listens attentively to Mr EJ's account of his current symptoms and displays empathy to its adverse impact on his life
   - understands his request for information on the natural history and possible treatments of campylobacter as the patient knows very little about this infection
   - uses his ideas about self-limiting illness in explanations
   - addresses his specific concerns about what to tell work and his expectations of when to resume air stewarding duties

9. *Give the patient the opportunity to be involved in significant management decisions*
   The doctor:
   - discusses the pros and cons of antibiotic and probiotic treatments and negotiates with the patient
   - encourages patient autonomy by providing him with enough information so that he feels able to discuss work issues with his company

Debrief

Discuss how the doctor could, if needed, improve his performance. In particular, assess whether the doctor:

- asked questions in a systematic and structured manner? If so, how?
- asked about red flag symptoms? If so, how long did this take? Was this sign-posted? (for example, did the doctor preface his questions with *"I need to ask some questions to rule out serious illness – do you have any of the following?"*)
- discussed the evidence base for appropriate treatments?
- provided appropriate occupational medicine advice?

If the consultation over-ran, did the doctor:

- take too long to ask the red flag questions?
- spend too much time on small-talk?
- attempt to reduce consulting time by offering the patient a face-to-face appointment instead? This option may not be the most efficient use of resources.

Revising data gathering

What questions could the doctor ask to discover the patient's ideas, concerns, expectations and health beliefs?

- Ideas: *"What, in your experience, has been the best way of dealing with food poisoning? What's worked, and not worked, for you in the past?"*
- Concerns: *"Is there anything in particular that concerns you about this positive campylobacter result?"*
- Expectations: *"It seems to me that we have discussed your symptoms and treatment. However, I suspect you may have some questions about work. Are there any questions in particular you'd like me to answer?"*
- Health beliefs: *"You suspect that because this is your second episode of gut infection, you may be predisposed to gut infections. Let's talk about this for a moment."*

Test your theoretical knowledge

For each of the following statements, answer true (T) or false (F).

Regarding food poisoning

1. Diarrhoea, cramping, abdominal pain, and fever within 24 hours of exposure to the organism are symptoms of campylobacteriosis.
2. The absence of symptoms excludes a diagnosis of campylobacteriosis.
3. Campylobacteriosis is often associated with the consumption of seafood, soft cheese, or untreated water.
4. The source of campylobacteriosis is often not found.
5. Microbiological examination of faeces is useful if there is a suspected public health hazard, e.g. diarrhoea in food handlers and healthcare workers.

6. Microbiological examination of faeces is useful if the patient is systemically unwell or has dysentery.
7. Loperamide is useful and safe in people with severe symptoms or dysentery.

Relevant literature

http://cks.library.nhs.uk/mobiledevices/ckscontent.aspx?rawurl=gastroenteritis

http://cks.library.nhs.uk/gastroenteritis/background_information/causitive_infections/campylobacter

Case 14 – Man with UTI

Brief to the doctor

Mr MN is a 24 year old man attending for the result of a urine test taken a week previously by your nurse practitioner.

Patient summary

Name	MN
Date of birth (Age)	24
Social and family history	Single Engineer
Past medical history	1 week ago – Nurse Practitioner Clinic: "*4/7 dysuria, frequency and urgency. Urine Prot tr, WBC +, Nit Pos. Send MSU. Trimethoprim 200mg bd 7/7. Pt will call me in 4d for result.*"
Current medication	None

Investigations

	1 week ago MSU:
WBC	$>10^7$/ml
RBC	Nil
Scanty mixed growth	?significance

Tasks for the doctor

In this case, the tasks are to:
- review the patient's response to treatment and relate this to the MSU result
- answer the patient's questions about how he developed a UTI

Brief to the patient – more about the patient

1. Profile:

- MN, a 24 year old engineering graduate, has worked for an international mining company since graduating 2 years ago
- shares a rented flat with his girlfriend, a nurse at the local hospital; they plan to get married next year and buy their own flat
- enjoys an active lifestyle and likes to keep fit and healthy
- he developed urinary symptoms just over a week ago, attended the nurse practitioner's minor illness clinic and was told he probably had a UTI. He was given a prescription for antibiotics and told to phone the nurse back for the result

2. He is seeing the doctor today because:

- he has some questions he would like to discuss, rather than phone as instructed:
  - he is concerned about how he developed a UTI
  - his symptoms have not changed with the antibiotics – does this mean the nurse got the diagnosis or treatment wrong?
- the frequency and urgency symptoms are causing a lot of disruption and embarrassment – he usually works on sites around the country and keeps having to find toilets in a hurry

3. Additional information:

- If the doctor asks specifically:
  - his work mates have teased him that he might have an STD. He has not noticed any symptoms. He has not had sex with anyone other than his girlfriend for the past 6 months. If he has an STD, does this mean his girlfriend has been unfaithful? His girlfriend is on the Pill; they do not use condoms.
  - while working in South Africa 8 months ago, he had unprotected sex with a secretary working in his company's offices in Cape Town. This continued over a 2 month period until he returned to the UK. He feels very guilty about this and has not told his girlfriend about it. Before returning to the UK, he went to a GU Medicine Clinic and had tests, including HIV, and was told he was clear.
- He wants the doctor to explain:
  - how UTIs are 'caught'
  - the MSU result
  - why the antibiotics given by the nurse practitioner have not worked
  - what other diagnoses are possible
  - whether other tests or treatments are required

- He had an episode of discharge when he was a student, but was treated and checked afterwards and told he was clear.
- If the doctor talks about HIV, Mr MN will want to discuss:
  - why another test is required as he was told he was clear in South Africa
  - the implications on insurance and getting a mortgage
  - the implications for his girlfriend and any children they might have
  - how and where the test will be done – he is concerned that someone at the hospital will recognise his name as he and his girlfriend know and socialise with a lot of the staff there
  - if the test was positive, how would the practice deal with this? Would staff be told about his status? How would the practice guarantee confidentiality?
  - if the test was positive, what treatment would he have to have and what are the success rates nowadays?
  - given his job travelling round the country and sometimes abroad, are there any restrictions or precautions he would have to take?
- If the doctor talks about chlamydia, Mr MN will want to discuss:
  - how it is caught
  - if he has it, does this mean his girlfriend has been unfaithful?
  - could the South African clinic have missed it?
  - if he caught it in South Africa, why has it only just started giving him symptoms, and why has his girlfriend not had any symptoms?
  - will his girlfriend need to be tested and how should he raise this with her?
- Mr MN prefers simple straightforward honest answers to questions and will repeat questions to the doctor if he feels the doctor is evading answering or not giving unequivocal answers. He would rather be told all the possibilities, however bad, than be kept in the dark.

Approach to be taken

A. Data gathering, examination and clinical assessment skills

1. *Define the clinical problem: clarify why the patient has presented today*
   The doctor:
   - reads the patient information provided prior to the consultation
   - asks open questions to explore:
     o Mr MN's response to treatment – *"How are you getting on?"*
     o his concerns over why he has not improved – *"What do you make of that?"*
     o any other issues concerning him – *"Is there anything else you are worried this might be?"*
   - empathises with Mr MN over the practical effects of his symptoms
   - asks closed questions to clarify details about the symptoms, past history, and sexual history
   - obtains a sexual history in order to assesses Mr MN's risk of HIV or STDs

2. *Performs an appropriate physical or mental examination*
   - In this case, an examination is not required.

B. Clinical management skills

3. *Make an appropriate working diagnosis*
   - The doctor, based on the history and MSU result should suspect chlamydia.
   - This is a clinically sound hypothesis and is an appropriate use of probability.
   - The doctor integrates information to raise the possibility of HIV.

4. *Explain the problem to the patient using appropriate language*
   The doctor:
   - having quickly established that Mr MN is intelligent and eager to understand his symptoms, addresses his agenda
   - explains the MSU result and the possibility of chlamydia infection
   - provides information on chlamydia, in particular, how it may be asymptomatic for some time
   - explains that specific tests need to be done for chlamydia and that his girlfriend will need to be tested
   - should adopt a patient-centred approach to ensure he addresses the patient's concerns and expectations
   - uses chunking and checking information – *"Before I move on, can I check that I have got things clear?"*

5. *Provide holistic care and use resources effectively*
   The doctor:
   - practises evidence-based medicine – there is a likelihood of chlamydia given the MSU result, and a possibility of HIV given the history of unprotected sex in a high-risk country
   - understands socioeconomic/cultural background – discusses ways of informing his girlfriend that she needs to be tested – "*Would you like to discuss how you might raise this matter with your girlfriend?*"
   - is able to discuss the benefits and other implications of HIV testing – including insurance, mortgage, future health and travel
   - provides Mr MN with verbal and written information on chlamydia and HIV

6. *Prescribe appropriately*
   The doctor:
   - advises Mr MN that a second HIV test is required before he can be told he is clear
   - does not prescribe antibiotics as the diagnosis is not certain and other STDs must be excluded
   - provides the patient with a referral letter to a GUM Clinic for investigation and consideration of HIV testing

7. *Specify the conditions and interval for follow-up*
   The doctor:
   - confirms understanding – "*Can I just check that I have explained things clearly – what is the plan for you?*"
   - signposts Mr MN to information on chlamydia and HIV and to GUM Clinics where he could be tested
   - offers a follow-up appointment to discuss any issues arising – safety netting

C. Interpersonal skills: know and treat this patient

8. *Achieve rapport*
   The doctor:
   - listens carefully to Mr MN's concerns about his symptoms not settling and the effects they have on him at work
   - without embarrassment, sympathetically and sensitively elicits Mr MN's past sexual history
   - places problem in psychosocial context – how it affects patient/girlfriend/work
   - understands his request for information on chlamydia
   - displays empathy when raising the question of whether Mr MN is at risk of HIV and should have another test
   - helps Mr MN explore ways of raising the issues with his girlfriend – "*Would you like to practise how you might tell her?*"

- answers Mr MN's questions using appropriate language
- is non-judgemental about Mr MN's past sexual experiences
- addresses the patient's specific concerns and expectations – *"Is there anything else you want to ask me?"*

9. *Give the patient the opportunity to be involved in significant management decisions*
The doctor:
- actively confirms the patient's understanding of the problem – *"Does this make sense to you?"*
- shares thoughts/involves patient – *"If I were to say that having unprotected sex in South Africa may have exposed you to HIV, what would you say?"*
- agrees balanced plans – *"Are you happy with this plan?"*

Debrief

This starts as a relatively straightforward clinical case; the real challenge is communication skills with the patient over the possibility of chlamydia, how he could have caught it and the implications on his relationship, and finally the issue of HIV. The ability to take a sexual history without being awkward or embarrassed is also tested.

Discuss how the doctor could, if needed, improve his performance. In particular, assess how the doctor:
- answered questions in language and style that satisfied Mr MN
- discussed the sensitive issues of infidelity, STDs and HIV
- developed empathy and trust
- managed time in the consultation – not wasting time gathering information at the expense of discussing the sensitive issues

Revising data gathering

What questions could the doctor ask to discover the patient's ideas, concerns, expectations and health beliefs?
- Ideas: "*You said that work colleagues have teased you about having an STD, could that be a possibility?*"
- Concerns: "*Would you like to discuss how chlamydia is caught and the range of symptoms it can cause?*"
- Expectations: "*The result of your urine test has not proven a normal infection; have you considered other possible causes?*"
- Health beliefs: "*You seem concerned that I am suggesting another HIV test even though you were given the 'all-clear' in South Africa, shall we talk about HIV testing?*"

Once the doctor has gathered sufficient information, how could he summarise the problem for the patient?
- Evaluate whether the doctor used appropriate language, paced his explanation, and whether the explanation was well organised and logical.

Test your theoretical knowledge

For each of the following statements, answer true (T) or false (F)
1. Approximately 20% of females infected with chlamydia are asymptomatic
2. *N. gonorrhoeaea* and *Chlamydia trachomatis* account for most cases of epididymitis in men under 35 years of age
3. Bacterial orchitis rarely occurs with an associated epididymitis and is usually bilateral
4. Untreated neonatal chlamydia conjunctivitis can result in blindness

5. A significant percentage of men and women with gonorrhoea also have pharyngitis, which is usually asymptomatic

Relevant literature

Rogstad KE, Palfreeman A, Rooney G, *et al.* (2006) *United Kingdom national guidelines on HIV testing*. London: Clinical Effectiveness Group, British Association of Sexual Health and HIV.

Chlamydia: www.emedicine.com/emerg/TOPIC925.HTM

Gonorrhoea: www.emedicine.com/emerg/TOPIC220.HTM

Orchitis: www.emedicine.com/emerg/TOPIC344.HTM

Case 15 – Childhood bedwetting

Brief to the doctor

Mrs DJ is a 29 year old woman who presents (without her 6 year old son) asking for advice on his bedwetting.

Patient summary

Name	Tomas J
Date of birth (Age)	6
Social and Family History	One sister, age 3
Past medical history	Healthy – achieved appropriate milestones for age
	Seen occasionally for mild, seasonal URTIs
Repeat medication	None

Tasks for the doctor

In this case, the tasks are to:
- clarify the extent and nature of the bedwetting
- the effect of the bedwetting on Tomas and his family
- provide evidence-based advice on treatments

Brief to the patient – more about the patient

1. Profile:

- Mrs DJ is 29 year old housewife; her husband is a car mechanic
- both her children are healthy and developing as expected
- Mrs DJ is worried about her 6 year old son's bedwetting

2. She is seeing the doctor today because:

- she is concerned that Tomas still wets the bed at least 2 times per week. He has never been dry at night, but he is dry during the day. He has no medical problems and does not suffer from constipation or urine infections.
- he is a lovely child who is achieving well at school; he has lots of friends
- she has declined the sleep-overs to which Tomas has been invited as she thinks it would be embarrassing for him if he bed-wets on a sleepover – she worries about him being teased
- now that her daughter is 3, she would like to leave her children with her mum for a week so that she and her husband can go on holiday, but the frequent changing and washing of bedding creates a burden of housework and she feels guilty approaching her 56 year old mother
- nobody in the family has had a bedwetting problem
- she has tried restricting drinks for Tomas at night but this has not made much difference
- she thought the problem would resolve by age 5, but Tomas is now 6. Does he have a problem predisposing him to bedwetting? Should he be investigated? Does he need tablet treatments? Is there anything else she should do?

3. Additional information:

- if the doctor refers her to the health visitor, she would like to know what she should expect in terms of assessment and advice?
- if the doctor mentions different options to her, she expects to be advised on the efficacy of each before deciding on what she would like for Tomas

Approach to be taken

A. Data gathering, examination and clinical assessment skills

1. Define the clinical problem: clarify why the patient has presented today
The doctor:
- notes from the patient information provided that this is a 6 year old with no significant past medical history
- asks mum open questions to explore the nature of the bedwetting (to make a diagnosis of primary nocturnal enuresis in a healthy, socially well adjusted 6 year old boy)
- asks what has made her present today (to discover that Mrs DJ is thinking of leaving the children with her mum for a week in the school holidays to have a break with her husband)
- asks closed questions to identify potentially reversible contributory factors: constipation, urinary tract infections, diet, stress (school problems / family discord / moving house), diabetes mellitus, ease of access to a toilet or potty, night lights, and bunk beds
- excludes red flags: neurological problems, behaviour problems, sleep apnoea
- elicits how the problem affects Tomas (embarrassment, social isolation, teasing by family members or friends)
- elicits how the problem affects the family (parental anxiety / frustration / punishment / extra work of laundry / effect of interrupted sleep)
- discovers her ideas that bedwetting should have ceased by age 6
- discovers her concerns about the social restriction (sleep-overs / family holidays)
- discovers her expectations for advice and a treatment plan

2. Performs an appropriate physical or mental examination
- In this case, an examination is not required. However, make arrangements to examine Tomas (abdomen, genitalia, spine (tuft of hair/lipoma), knee jerks, and a dipstick urinalysis).

B. Clinical management skills

3. Make an appropriate working diagnosis
- The doctor, based on the history, makes a working diagnosis of childhood primary nocturnal enuresis. There are no contributory factors.

4. Explain the problem to the patient using appropriate language
The doctor:
- contextualises the problem: 1 in 50 7 year olds wet the bed more than once a week and 15% get better without treatment each year. Children who are passing large volumes at night may not be producing sufficient

anti-diuretic hormone (ADH); small volumes may indicate small, irritable bladders; or the child may be sleeping so deeply that he is unaware of the sensation of a full bladder.

- having established the absence of red flags and contributory factors, provides general support and advice: signposting to ERIC (enuresis resource and information centre), using waterproof mattress coverings, avoiding caffeine after 3 pm, timing and amount of fluid intake
- refers to the health visitor for specific advice: star charts to reward getting out of bed to use the toilet, or enuresis alarms (bed or body-worn) for the child to learn to stop urinating when the alarm sounds – because they require the child's cooperation, alarms are usually reserved for children over 7 years
- advises Mrs DJ that drug treatment, with imipramine or desmopressin, is appropriate for short periods such a sleep-overs or holidays away from home; both drugs can be used in a 6 year old, and are effective while taken but bedwetting recurs on discontinuation

5. *Provide holistic care and use resources effectively*
   The doctor:
   - practises evidence-based medicine that is informed by national or local guidelines (www.cks.nhs.uk/bedwetting_enuresis/evidence/references#-477798)
   - involves the health visitor in on-going treatment and support
   - does not refer to secondary care in the absence of red flags and contributory symptoms

6. *Prescribe appropriately*
   The doctor:
   - is aware of the indications and side-effects of imipramine and desmopressin
   - discusses prescription but is unlikely to prescribe without having examined the child and organised urine tests first

7. *Specify the conditions and interval for follow-up*
   The doctor:
   - signposts Mrs DJ to information on nocturnal enuresis, such as www.eric.org.uk/
   - arranges urinalysis
   - offers a follow-up appointment to examine Tomas, discuss urine test findings, and review the problem

C. Interpersonal skills: know and treat this patient

8. *Achieve rapport*
   The doctor:
   - listens attentively to Mrs DJ's concerns regarding the continued bedwetting and its impact on the family
   - displays empathy to the workload and financial burden the bedwetting creates
   - addresses the patient's specific expectations about a long-term solution and what to do for sleep-overs and holidays
   - is sensitive in his queries regarding the parents' frustration and the possible punishment of the child

9. *Give the patient the opportunity to be involved in significant management decisions*
   The doctor:
   - shares his thoughts, for example, *"I am reassured by what you have told me about Tomas's physical and social development. I think this problem will resolve in time as his hormones and bladder mature. There are a few things we could do to help Tomas. I'll give you the options first and then you can tell me which you'd like to try."*
   - encourages autonomy and opinions – provides her with information so she feels able to choose the most appropriate option for Tomas and the family

Debrief

Discuss how the doctor could, if needed, improve his performance. In particular, assess whether the doctor:

- structured the history taking? For example, did the doctor preface his questions with *"I need to ask some questions to rule out serious illness – does Tomas have any of the following?"*
- assessed the impact of the bedwetting on the entire family? If so, how?
- addressed Mrs DJ's specific concerns? If so, how?
- made appropriate use of resources?
- outlined the reasons for follow-up?

If the consultation over-ran, did the doctor:

- ask open rather than closed questions when assessing contributory and red flag symptoms?
- provide overly detailed explanations of each option?
- signpost inadequately, that is, duplicate the services of the health visitor (or continence advisor) in providing detailed information and on-going support?

Revising data gathering

What questions could the doctor ask to discover the patient's ideas, concerns, expectations and health beliefs?

- Ideas: *"What is your understanding of bedwetting – causes, treatments and so on?"*
- Concerns: *"Is there anything in particular about the current situation that is worrying you?"*
- Expectations: *"When you came to see me today, was there anything in particular you'd hoped I'd do for you?"*
- Health beliefs: *"You seem concerned that your 6 year old hasn't achieved night-time dryness. Let's talk about this for a moment."*

Test your theoretical knowledge

For each of the following statements, answer true (T) or false (F).

Regarding childhood nocturnal enuresis

1. Enuresis is the involuntary discharge of urine by day or night or both, in a child aged 6 years or older, in the absence of congenital or acquired defects of the nervous system or urinary tract.
2. Up to one-third of parents become intolerant of the enuresis and consequently also of their child.
3. 10% of children with nocturnal enuresis have a positive family history of childhood bedwetting.
4. The treatment of chronic constipation leads to the resolution of nocturnal enuresis in two-thirds of affected children.

5. The odds ratio of enuresis in children with ADHD is 2.7 times higher than in controls.
6. Cola and chocolate are diuretics.
7. The only investigation required in primary nocturnal enuresis is urinalysis to exclude diabetes mellitus and a urinary tract infection.
8. Restrict fluids such that the child has about six small drinks a day, spaced out throughout the day, the last one 2 hours before bed.
9. Sharing a room is a relative contra-indication to the use of an enuresis alarm.
10. Desmopressin and imipramine are of equal efficacy.

Relevant literature

www.cks.nhs.uk/bedwetting_enuresis/evidence/references#-477798

Case 16 – Prostate cancer

Brief to the doctor

Mr OP is a 74 year old man who saw a locum 4 days ago because of urinary symptoms. The locum arranged tests for MSU, FBC, U&Es, LFTs and PSA. Mr OP attends today for the results.

Patient summary

Name	OP
Date of birth (Age)	74
Social and family history	Married Retired carpenter and joiner No FH CVD
Past medical history	4 days ago – Locum: *"Frequency, nocturia ×4, dribbling. Urine NAD. Abdo NAD. RE hard nodular left lobe prostate. Check bloods and review prior to referral. Pt not told prostate feels suspicious."*
Current medication	None

Investigations

4 days ago:

Hb	11.2 g/dl (12–15)
MCV	78.4 (83–105)
WBC	2.3 (4–11)
ESR	84
Na	130 (135–145)
K	3.4 (3.5–5)
Urea	5.6 (2.5–6.7)
Creatinine	76 (70–150)
AlkP	185 (95–280)
AST	28
ALT	31 (10–45)
PSA	10 (<4.0)

Tasks for the doctor

In this case, the tasks are to:

- review results and the locum's clinical findings
- explain the results and the necessary actions to the patient
- deal with the patient's anxiety over the possible diagnosis

Brief to the patient – more about the patient

1. Profile:

- Mr OP is a 74 year old retired carpenter and joiner
- he likes to keeps active, although after a hip replacement 4 years ago he has not been as active as he hoped he would be
- he has been troubled with increasing frequency, nocturia and dribbling stream for the past year, but things have got worse over the past 2 months
- he feels well in himself, but gets tired easily – he attributes this to his age
- he does not like to make a fuss and believes doctors should not be questioned – they are experts and he should take their advice

2. He is seeing the doctor today because:

- the locum doctor took some tests and told him to come back to see one of the regular doctors for the results
- a lot of his friends have prostate problems and are taking tablets that help; he expects the doctor is going to start him on these today

3. Additional information:

- If the doctor asks specifically:
  - symptoms – nocturia ×4, frequency by day every 60–90 minutes, weak stream with terminal dribbling; no blood seen
  - he has not lost any weight and has no other symptoms
  - his father's brother died of prostate cancer. His father died of old age. His uncle was treated by orchidectomy – Mr OP is horrified at this treatment.
- If the doctor suggests that the results are suspicious or that referral for more tests is required, Mr OP will ask if there is a possibility of cancer.
- He is still sexually active.
- His wife had a small heart attack 2 years ago, but is well and active now. He tries not to trouble her with things because she is a worrier and he is concerned that worrying will strain her heart.
- He has two children who both live locally and visit regularly.
- He has not considered the possibility of having cancer because he feels well, unlike his uncle who was ill and lost a lot of weight.
- If the doctor mentions cancer:
  - he will get very anxious about his wife, possible treatments and prognosis
  - he will want the doctor to explain what treatments are possible and their success
  - he will want to discuss what he should tell his wife and whether it will affect her heart

Approach to be taken

A. Data gathering, examination and clinical assessment skills

1. *Define the clinical problem: clarify why the patient has presented today*
   The doctor:
   - reads the patient information provided prior to the consultation
   - asks open questions to explore what the locum told Mr OP and what Mr OP suspects might be the cause of his symptoms: "*Can you tell me what the locum said to you?*" and "*What do you think might be the cause?*"
   - asks closed questions to clarify Mr OP's symptoms and family history
   - responds to non-verbal cues: "*You look like you weren't expecting to be told you needed to be referred, am I right?*"

2. *Performs an appropriate physical or mental examination*
   - In this case, an examination is not required.

B. Clinical management skills

3. *Make an appropriate working diagnosis*
   - The doctor integrates information from the history, the locum's examination and blood results and makes a working diagnosis of suspected prostatic cancer.

4. *Explain the problem to the patient using appropriate language*
   The doctor:
   - informs Mr OP that the blood test results and the locum's examination are not normal and that further tests at the hospital are indicated
   - uses a patient-centred approach to address Mr OP's concerns and expectations – "*I cannot say whether this is cancer or not until you have had some tests at the hospital*"
   - checks the patient's understanding: "*This has been a bit of a shock for you, can I just go over what we have just talked about before moving on to the next bit?*"
   - provides some information on what tests may be required, and what treatments are available: transrectal ultrasound, biopsy, bone scans, treatments depend on stage and assessed risk and range from active surveillance only through surgery to radiotherapy and chemo- and hormone therapy

5. *Provide holistic care and use resources effectively*
   The doctor:
   - practises evidence-based medicine and is informed by national or local guidelines – NICE (2008) *Prostate cancer: diagnosis and treatment*

- allows Mr OP time to explore his anxieties about telling his wife his possible diagnosis
- provides Mr OP with information if required

6. *Prescribe appropriately*
The doctor:
- is aware of national and local guidelines:
  - for suspected cancer referrals: NICE (2005) *Referral guidelines for suspected cancer* (CG27 – www.nice.org.uk/Guidance/CG27)
  - for prostate cancer: NICE (2008) *Prostate cancer: diagnosis and treatment* (CG58 – www.nice.org.uk/Guidance/CG58)

7. *Specify the conditions and interval for follow-up*
The doctor:
- offers a follow-up appointment to discuss any issues arising from his outpatient attendance or if Mr OP has any questions or concerns
- safety netting – "*You should have received an appointment to be seen within the next 2 weeks; let me know if you have heard nothing in one week's time*"
- arranges to see Mr OP after the hospital appointment

C. Interpersonal skills: know and treat this patient

8. *Achieve rapport*
The doctor:
- sensitively informs Mr OP about the need for referral
- explores and clarifies Mr OP's concerns and expectations: "*You look concerned. Is there anything particular worrying you?*"
- listens attentively to Mr OP's concerns about his wife
- displays empathy: "*I understand why you are worried about the effect this might have on your wife; would you like to discuss this for a while?*"

9. *Give the patient the opportunity to be involved in significant management decisions*
The doctor:
- actively confirms the patient's understanding of the problem: "*What does all this mean to you?*"
- provides the patient with information by answering his questions, but does not raise unnecessary alarm as the diagnosis has not been confirmed
- supports the patient by discussing his concerns about possible treatments (particularly orchidectomy) and how to tell his wife

Debrief

This case focuses on the doctor's ability to raise the possibility of bad news.

Discuss how the doctor could, if needed, improve his performance. In particular, assess how the doctor:
- managed time in the consultation – did s/he spend too much time reviewing symptoms and not enough on answering Mr OP's concerns?
- raised the need for further tests and answered Mr OP's question about whether or not he had cancer

Revising data gathering

What questions could the doctor ask to discover the patient's ideas, concerns, expectations and health beliefs?
- Ideas: *"I understand that you wouldn't want the same treatment your uncle had; do you know anything about other treatments?"*
- Concerns: *"I understand that cancer is a frightening word, would you like to discuss prostate cancer in more detail?"*
- Expectations: *"I am going to refer you to the hospital; would you like me to outline what tests they are likely to want to do?"*
- Health beliefs: *"You are worried that this might affect your wife's health; would you like to spend some time talking about this?"*

Test your theoretical knowledge

For each of the following statements, answer true (T) or false (F).
1. Serum PSA level alone is a poor predictor of the presence of prostate cancer
2. Risk factors include diets high in red meats and fat
3. An affected first degree relative triples the relative risk
4. In low risk men, radical treatment may be deferred until there is evidence of progression of the cancer
5. Hormonal therapy is routinely offered to all men with intermediate or high risk of localised prostate cancer

Relevant literature

UK Prostate Link: www.prostate-link.org.uk

Cancer Research UK: www.cancerresearchuk.org

A framework for breaking bad news: www.skillscascade.com/badnews.htm

DoH (2003) Breaking Bad News... Regional Guidelines. *Department of Health, Social Services and Public Safety, Northern Ireland Group of the National Council for Hospice and Specialist Palliative care*: www.dhsspsni.gov.uk

Fallon M. (1998) ABC of palliative care: Communication with patients, families and other professionals. *BMJ,* **316**: 130–132.

Maguir GP. (1999) Breaking bad news: explaining cancer diagnosis and prognosis. *MJA,* **171**: 288–289.

Case 17 – Painful calf

Brief to the doctor

Mrs RD is a 29 year old woman who presents with a painful left calf.

Patient summary

Name	RD
Date of birth (Age)	29
Social and Family History	Married, no children Teacher Non-smoker
Past medical history	Difficulty sleeping (1 year ago) – given zopiclone Cervical smear 5 years ago – normal
Repeat medication	None
Tests	Values are from 6 months ago
BMI	24.2
BP	118/72
	Value from 1 year ago
PHQ score	6/27

Tasks for the doctor

In this case, the tasks are to:
- clarify whether Mrs RD's fears about having a DVT are well-founded
- negotiate appropriate and timely investigation
- explain the nature of the investigation(s) in simple, jargon-free language

Brief to the patient – more about the patient

1. Profile:

- Mrs RD is a 29 year old woman who works as a teacher in the local primary school
- when she married 4 months ago, she stopped taking the combined oral contraceptive pill (Microgynon) which she had used, without problems, since the age of 19; she hopes to get pregnant and her period is 2 days late – she has not done a pregnancy test as yet

2. She is seeing the doctor today because:

- her left calf has been painful for 36 hours – it feels swollen and warm to the touch
- she drove down from Edinburgh to London 3 days ago; there were problems on the road and the journey took 11 hours, but there was no opportunity during the 3 hour delay to leave the car
- she does not have a past history of deep vein thrombosis (DVT), is no longer on Microgynon, and has not had recent surgery. Her sister (aged 28) had a DVT during the 20th week of her pregnancy. Nobody else in the family has had a DVT or pulmonary embolus (PE).
- she has not done any recent strenuous physical exercise, nor does she feel unwell in herself

3. Additional information:

- Mrs RD is worried that she may be pregnant and she may have a DVT
- she expects a referral to the hospital for a scan
- her sister was given injections to treat the DVT – will she be put on injections too? She has needle-phobia and does not believe that she will manage to self-inject.

Approach to be taken

A. Data gathering, examination and clinical assessment skills

1. *Define the clinical problem: clarify why the patient has presented today*
   The doctor:
   - reads the patient information provided prior to the consultation
   - asks open questions to explore the nature and duration of the symptoms
   - empathises with Mrs RD's concerns that this may be a DVT
   - asks closed questions to assess whether the patient is at high risk for DVT: previous history of DVT, recent surgery, recent immobility, malignancy?
   - asks about PE symptoms: shortness or breath, pleuritic chest pain, haemoptysis?
   - works through the diagnostic sieve to rule out other possible causes of a painful calf, such as cellulitis, lymphangitis, muscle strain, a ruptured Baker's cyst, or venous insufficiency. The doctor could sign-post his systematic questioning of the differential diagnosis by prefacing his questions with: *"I need to ask some questions to rule out all the possible causes of a sore calf – do you have any of the following symptoms: a red rash on the calf, feeling unwell in yourself, muscle strain from sport or an injury?"*.
   - asks about the possibility of pregnancy, an important red flag
   - discovers Mrs RD's idea that she has a DVT, her concern that she will need to treat the DVT by self injecting, her expectation of a referral to hospital for a scan and her belief that DVTs are treated by subcutaneous heparin

2. *Performs an appropriate physical or mental examination*
   - An examination is required and should be guided by the Wells scoring system – see www.bradfordvts.co.uk/WEBLINKS/consultation%20tools/wells%20score%20for%20DVTs.html or www.medscape.com/viewarticle/520153_appendix2
   - Look for:
     - tenderness along entire deep vein system
     - swelling of entire leg
     - measure the calf circumference 10 cm below the tibial tuberosity and look for >3 cm difference in calf circumference
     - pitting oedema confined to the symptomatic leg
     - collateral dilated superficial veins (non-varicose)
     - the absence of signs pointing to an alternative diagnosis, such as cellulitis, congestive cardiac failure, muscle sprains or a Baker's cyst
   - In this patient, assume the only sign present is moderate tenderness (4/10) in the posterior aspect of the left calf which is worse when the patient stands up or when you passively dorsiflex her ankle.

B. Clinical management skills

3. *Make an appropriate working diagnosis*
   - The doctor, based on the history and examination, makes a working diagnosis of DVT. If the patient is not pregnant, the risk is low and a D-dimer test should be done. If the patient is pregnant, the risk is moderate to high and an ultrasound scan should be organised.

4. *Explain the problem to the patient using appropriate language*
   The doctor:
   - having clarified that Mrs RD has a good idea of what a DVT is based on her sister's experience, addresses her agenda
   - explains that further investigation (blood test or ultrasound scan) depends on whether or not she is pregnant – the doctor organises a pregnancy test
   - addresses her idea that she has a DVT. She may have a DVT, but further investigation is needed before a diagnosis can be made. Only 50% of patients with classic signs of a DVT actually have one.
   - Addresses her concerns: she is worried about self-injecting subcutaneous heparin. If she is pregnant and has a DVT (two assumptions at present), subcutaneous heparin is needed. If she is not pregnant and has a DVT, a brief period of subcutaneous injection is followed by oral warfarin therapy. The fact that injections are subcutaneous (rather than intramuscular) and may only be needed for a brief period may be reassuring to the patient.
   - Addresses her expectations: a scan is needed only if her pregnancy test is positive, or if her D-dimer result is positive.

5. *Provide holistic care and use resources effectively*
   The doctor:
   - practises evidence-based medicine
   - is informed by national or local guidelines (http://cks.library.nhs.uk/deep_vein_thrombosis/management)

6. *Prescribe appropriately*
   The doctor:
   - is aware of national and local guidelines
   - does not prescribe until further information is available

7. *Specify the conditions and interval for follow-up*
   The doctor:
   - arranges for a pregnancy test. If positive, arranges for a scan. If negative, arranges for a D-dimer test.
   - if DVT is suspected on clinical grounds, further assessment and definitive diagnosis on the day of presentation is ideal

C. Interpersonal skills: know and treat this patient

8. *Achieve rapport*
   The doctor:
   - listens attentively to Mrs RD's concerns about having a DVT
   - understands her request for an ultrasound scan and deals with the request appropriately and with sensitivity
   - gently challenges or corrects the patient's assumption that she has a DVT requiring treatment with subcutaneous heparin

9. *Give the patient the opportunity to be involved in significant management decisions*
   The doctor:
   - negotiates with the patient when the pregnancy test will be done
   - gives the patient sufficient information to appreciate that time is of the essence and definitive testing should be completed within 24 hours of presentation

Debrief

Discuss how the doctor could, if needed, improve his performance. In particular, assess whether the doctor:

- took a systematic history, quickly eliciting the risk factors for DVT, and working through the diagnostic sieve
- discussed and prioritised the order of the investigations, while addressing the patient's expectation of a scan appropriately
- explained the investigations (D-dimer testing) in simple language

If the consultation over-ran, was the doctor:

- systematic in his history taking – were questions asked without appropriate signposting?
- systematic, thorough and confident in his examination technique?
- logical and organised in arranging further investigation and follow-up?

Revising data gathering

What questions could the doctor ask to discover the patient's ideas, concerns, expectations and health beliefs?

- Ideas: *"What do you imagine the treatment for DVT will be?"*
- Concerns: *"With regard to DVTs, what are you most worried about?"*
- Expectations: *"How was your sister's DVT diagnosed? Did you also expect to be scanned?"*
- Health beliefs: *"You have good grounds for suspecting a DVT. Let's just talk about how we go about confirming or disproving a DVT."*

Test your theoretical knowledge

For each of the following statements, answer true (T) or false (F).

Regarding DVT and PE

1. Dyspnoea, chest pain, or haemoptysis are symptoms of DVT.
2. A positive Homan's sign is pain in the calf on active abrupt, forceful dorsiflexion of the ankle with the leg outstretched (knee extended).
3. The D-dimer assay is a test for the presence of fibrin degradation products in plasma, which are raised in DVT.
4. Pregnancy raises plasma levels of D-dimer.
5. D-dimer assays are less sensitive for proximal than distal DVT.
6. D-dimer levels are unaffected by heparin.
7. Moderate to high risk patients, with a positive D-dimer test and a negative ultrasound, do not require repeat ultrasonography.
8. One of the differential diagnoses of a DVT is a ruptured Baker's cyst, which is a cyst that forms in the ankle from an outpouching of synovial membrane of the ankle joint.

Relevant literature

http://cks.library.nhs.uk/deep_vein_thrombosis/management

www.youtube.com/watch?v=Y2XHP-aaDpc – presentation on DVT by Stephen Bright

http://onlinelibrary.wiley.com/doi/10.1046/j.1365-2141.2003.04723.x/full

Case 18 – Leg ulcer

Brief to the doctor

Miss QR is an 85 year old lady who is usually seen regularly in surgery by your senior partner (Dr Smith). She has requested a home visit because she has knocked her leg and it is 'leaking water'.

Patient summary

Name	QR
Date of birth (Age)	85
Social and family history	Lives alone in privately owned old people's flat Warden on site
Past medical history	Hypertension – 30 years Leg oedema – 4 years Osteoarthritis both knees – 15 years Obesity – 45 years
	Saw Dr Smith 1 month ago: "*No great change. BP 140/84, oedema to just above knees. Walking with a stick. Blood test done. No change in medication.*"
Current medication	Lisinopril 20 mg daily Furosemide 40 mg twice daily
Investigations	1 month ago – FBC, U&Es and fasting glucose all normal

Tasks for the doctor

In this case, the tasks are to:
- explore and clarify Miss QR's concerns
- formulate an appropriate clinical and social management plan, utilising other members of the PCT

Brief to the patient – more about the patient

1. Profile:

- Miss QR is an 85 year old lady who lives alone in a privately owned old flat in an old people's block with a resident warden
- she has long-standing hypertension and osteoarthritis in her knees. She has been overweight most of her life and knows she should lose weight, but has no motivation to do so. For the past 4 years her legs have been swollen and this is limiting her mobility significantly.
- she attends surgery every 3 months for a check with Dr Smith
- she has no family history of CVD or DM

2. She is seeing the doctor today because:

- she knocked her leg on the corner of a coffee table last week, causing a superficial wound which she put a plaster on initially, but she started to leak fluid from the wound and when she removed the plaster she tore off skin, leaving a superficial raw area
- the leg has continued to leak. Friends have bought dressings and bandages from the local chemist who has now suggested to them that she should be seen. She has to sit with plastic bags under her leg to prevent the carpet getting soiled and has had to put a waterproof mattress cover on her bed. She is very meticulous about hygiene and finds the leaking fluid repugnant.
- she is terrified of developing leg ulcers
- she is very proud that her blood tests for kidney function, diabetes and cholesterol have always been normal and feels that this justifies her belief that there would be no real benefit to her if she lost weight
- she feels well despite the current problem

3. Additional information:

- If the doctor asks specifically:
  - she lives on the first floor, but there is a lift
  - she has been elevating her legs on a low stool
- She will not accept hospital admission unless she is very ill.
- She has a home help who visits once weekly to clean and do her shopping. Miss QR can cook for herself and is completely independent.
- She believes a District Nurse should be asked to visit and dress her leg.
- She is struggling to cope with her single stick and believes a frame might be a better option; she is reluctant to ask for this as she feels she is being over-demanding when resources in the NHS are scarce.
- If the doctor examines her:

System	Examination findings
General	No pallor. Grossly overweight.
CVS	HR 76 SR. HS 1+2 +nil. BP 136/82 Lungs clear Pitting oedema to mid-thigh level Unable to palpate pedal pulses due to oedema
Abdo	No mass. No organomegaly. No ascites.
Legs	Oedema as noted OA knees with valgus deformity on right 4 × 4cm superficial ulcer left shin. Very thin shiny surrounding skin with some small scattered vesicles. No surrounding cellulitis and no slough on ulcer. No evidence of infection. Serous fluid leaking from ulcer.

Approach to be taken

A. Data gathering, examination and clinical assessment skills

1. *Define the clinical problem: clarify why the patient has presented today*
   The doctor:
   - reads the patient information provided prior to the consultation
   - asks open questions to explore why she has asked for a home visit a week after injuring her leg – *"Have you any thoughts about what can be done to help you?"*
   - empathises with her about the leaking fluid
   - asks closed questions to clarify details about her past history and current medication, and her general health at present

2. *Performs an appropriate physical or mental examination*
   - Explains that an examination is required using appropriate language.
   - Performs a targeted examination to assess wound and degree of heart failure – this should include looking at the wound, assessing the extent of her oedema, checking JVP and listening to her heart and lungs.
   - Examination addresses patient's concerns – to see whether she has an ulcer.

B. Clinical management skills

3. *Make an appropriate working diagnosis*
   - The doctor, based on the history and examination, makes a working diagnosis of leg ulcer in a lady with heart failure.

4. *Explain the problem to the patient using appropriate language*
   The doctor:
   - explains why the ulcer has developed and why it has continued to leak fluid
   - addresses the patient's concerns and expectations – *"There is a good chance we can get the ulcer to heal as it is shallow, but we will need to decrease your leg swelling to help this happen."*

5. *Provide holistic care and use resources effectively*
   The doctor:
   - arranges for the District Nurse to visit to assess the ulcer and provide appropriate dressings and monitor response
   - explains what the District Nurse is likely to do – Doppler Ankle Brachial Pressure Index (ABPI)
   - provides some information on what Miss QR can do to help herself – good skin care, low salt intake, importance of mobility and exercise, leg elevation when immobile
   - identifies the social (decreased mobility) and psychological (finds the leaking fluid repugnant) impact of this diagnosis on Miss QR

- uses PCT and other resources – District Nurse and physiotherapy/OT assessment of whether a frame might enable safer mobility than her current stick

6. *Prescribe appropriately*
   The doctor:
   - decides to see if rest and elevation will be beneficial before altering treatment
   - decides to await the result of the ABPI before formulating an ulcer management plan

7. *Specify the conditions and interval for follow-up*
   The doctor:
   - offers a follow-up appointment either with him/herself or with Dr Smith to monitor progress
   - confirms understanding – *"Is there anything I haven't explained or you don't understand?"*

C. Interpersonal skills: know and treat this patient

8. *Achieve rapport*
   The doctor:
   - explores and clarifies Miss QR's concerns – *"Is there anything in particular you are worried about?"*
   - places problem in psychosocial context – *"How are you coping with all this on your own?"*
   - supports the long relationship Miss QR has with Dr Smith
   - addresses the patient's specific concerns and expectations – District Nurse visit and provision of a frame

9. *Give the patient the opportunity to be involved in significant management decisions*
   The doctor:
   - actively confirms patient's understanding of the problem – *"Have I adequately explained to you why your leg is leaking fluid?"*
   - uses time as a therapeutic tool – no medication change, monitor effects of ulcer treatment and elevation
   - encourages autonomy and opinions – *"Have you had any thoughts on what I can do to help?"*
   - supports and congratulates her in looking after the ulcer initially and preventing infection

Debrief

Discuss how the doctor could, if needed, improve his performance. In particular, assess how the doctor:
- established rapport with a patient who usually saw another doctor
- explored Miss QR's concerns and beliefs
- explained the possible management plans that may result from the ABPI results

Revising data gathering

What questions could the doctor ask to discover the patient's ideas, concerns, expectations and health beliefs?
- Ideas: "*Why do you think the wound has not healed as quickly as you expected?*"
- Concerns: "*Is there anything you are particularly worried about?*"
- Expectations: "*You have done really well to keep the wound clean, but it isn't healing as you expected. What do you think needs to be done now?*"
- Health beliefs: "*The pharmacist advised getting the wound checked – let's discuss wound healing briefly.*"

Test your theoretical knowledge

For each of the following statements, answer true (T) or false (F).
1. The cause of most leg ulcers is unclear
2. A past history of cigarette smoking, phlebitis and previous trauma should always be taken
3. Skin pigmentation, shiny hairless skin and varicose veins suggest an arterial cause
4. ABPI measurements in patients with diabetes may not be reliable
5. Ulcers should be scrubbed clean to remove all debris and exudate
6. Graduated compression bandages should be used to control oedema
7. Patients with an ABPI <0.5 require urgent referral
8. Ulcers should be swabbed routinely so that any infection can be identified and treated promptly

Relevant literature

www.sign.ac.uk/guidelines/fulltext/120/index.html

www.worldwidewounds.com/2001/march/Vowden/Doppler-assessment-and-ABPI.html

www.cks.nhs.uk/leg_ulcer_venous/management/detailed_answers/interpreting_doppler_studies

Case 19 – A list of symptoms

Brief to the doctor

Mrs SW is a 52 year old woman who presents with a list of problems:

1. pain in right calf
2. voice is hoarse
3. I had recent blood tests – what are the results?
4. I think I'm going through the menopause – feeling low, tired, no sex drive, weight gain

Patient summary

Name	SW
Date of birth (Age)	52
Social and Family History	Married for 28 years with one child (27) Works from home providing IT support
Past medical history	Sleep disorders (8 months ago) – issued zopiclone Right leg sciatica (8 months ago) – issued analgesia Voice hoarseness (3 years ago) – no abnormalities found by ENT; assumed related to gastric reflux Intermittent asthma (from teenager)
Repeat medication	Diprobase 500 g as directed (AD) Seretide 125 evohaler Cfc-free 100 µg / puff (AD) Ventolin evohaler Cfc-free 100 µg / puff (AD) Lansoprazole 30 mg once daily × 28

Consultation note by Dr Brown (4 weeks ago):

'Voice hoarseness: has had previous episodes and investigations by ENT in the past. No evidence of cancer and felt related to gastric reflux. Gargles after using steroid inhalers. Has been having more reflux symptoms lately despite cutting down alcohol dramatically from 50 units per week and changing diet. Last week, only had 4 glasses of wine in total. O/E: no cervical lymph nodes felt. Throat OK. Chest clear. No creps or wheeze. Plan: Trial of doubling PPI. Get bloods for general health screen. Review thereafter.'

Blood tests   Tests were done two weeks ago
   Hb   12.5 g/dl (12–15)
   MCV   102 (83–105)
   Liver functions tests   normal
   Renal function   normal
   TSH   4.32 (0.35–5.5)
   Fasting glucose   6.2 (3–5.5)
   Total cholesterol   5.7
   HDL   1.1
   H. pylori   negative

Tasks for the doctor

In this case, the tasks are to:

- negotiate the problem list, prioritising appropriately
- discuss the blood results, especially the abnormal fasting glucose
- discuss the menopausal symptoms
- establish that the calf pain and hoarse voice are long-standing problems, without recent red-flags, and agree review of these issues at follow-up appointments

Brief to the patient – more about the patient

1. Profile:

- Mrs SW is a 52 year old woman who has worked from home for the last 6 months. She misses the social interaction of working in an office environment and now feels lonely and low.
- she is happily married; her husband has noticed the increased alcohol consumption, which she has attributed to helping her sleep at night
- Mrs SW doesn't see the doctor often and because she is worried about her health, she presents with a list of symptoms. The list also helps her to remember what she wants to discuss. She is getting forgetful these days, a sign of the menopause, she thinks.

2. She is seeing the doctor today because:

- she has had an intermittent dull pain (3/10) in her right calf, worse on standing up from gardening, since her sciatica 8 months ago. The pain does not interrupt sleep, but is an irritating niggle that rarely interferes with everyday activities. She wants to know if she should continue with the exercises the physiotherapist gave her, or whether she needs to see the physiotherapist again for further assessment and treatment.
- she still has an intermittent hoarse voice, but things are much better. Dr Brown spoke to her about reducing her alcohol intake and taking lansoprazole 30 mg for 1 month. This has helped but she has run out of tablets. A repeat script is required but she doesn't know if she should take 15 mg or 30 mg of lansoprazole now.
- she had blood tests done. Dr Brown wanted to check that she was not anaemic or diabetic or had thyroid problems, possible causes of her tiredness. She does not believe she has these conditions. Dr Brown wanted the other tests as 'a general health screen in the over 40s'. When told about the raised fasting glucose, she is adamant that she had fasted, and she is surprised and slightly worried by the result: what does it mean, and what does she need to do about it? She does not have symptoms of DM. No one in her family has DM.
- she is worried about her menopausal symptoms: feeling low, tired, no sex drive, weight gain and irregular periods for the last 4 months. Flushing occurs, but infrequently, so this is not a major issue. Mrs SW feels she lacks the energy to exercise, socialize, and make more friends. If she socialized more, she'd not drink at home during the evening. She wants to get her energy back.
- she attributes her lack of energy to the menopause – her 'idea'
- she is concerned about getting a DVT from HRT seeing that she already has a 'weak calf'

- she expects to be told about the pros and cons of HRT; she does not expect a prescription for HRT today, but she does expect a prescription for lansoprazole

3. Additional information:

- if the doctor offers her a prescription for HRT, she says she'd like to read up on it first. She'd also like to consider alternatives such as St John's Wort or valerian for sleep. She expects the doctor to signpost her to suitable information.

4. *Explain the problem to the patient using appropriate language*
    The doctor:
    - explains that a diagnosis should not be made from a single blood test – the doctor organises a GTT, appropriately refers to the phlebotomist and gives clear instructions to the patient
    - provides information on the treatment of peri-menopausal symptoms: indicates that HRT may increase energy levels, SSRIs may help with flushing and valerian may help sleep; St John's wort is an enzyme inducer and may interfere with prescribed medication
    - explains the risks and benefits of HRT in appropriate language, and addresses the patient's particular concern regarding the risk of DVT on HRT
    - checks the patient's understanding at each point – if understanding is good, the doctor moves forward to the next item on the patient's list
    - prescribes an appropriate dose of lansoprazole for one month and negotiates review
    - negotiates review of the calf pain, explaining that a thorough reassessment of the sciatica and calf pain is required prior to making a decision regarding referral to physiotherapy. Alternatively, if the physiotherapy department had offered the patient an open-access appointment on discharge, she could call them directly for advice.

5. *Provide holistic care and use resources effectively*
    The doctor:
    - prioritises the issues effectively
    - makes balanced plans which are either doctor- or patient-centred as appropriate; for example, dealing with the raised fasting glucose is doctor-centred and dealing with the peri-menopausal symptoms is patient-centred
    - discusses conventional and complementary medicines, if Mrs SW is interested in the latter, for the treatment of her peri-menopausal symptoms; advice follows national or local guidelines (http://cks.library.nhs.uk/menopause)

6. *Prescribe appropriately*
    The doctor:
    - is aware of national and local guidelines (http://cks.library.nhs.uk/dyspepsia_proven_gord)
    - checks the patient's understanding of the medication and the amounts of medication required

7. *Specify the conditions and interval for follow-up*
    The doctor:
    - signposts Mrs SW to information on the menopause
    - offers a follow-up appointment to discuss issues not dealt with today; in particular, review of the voice hoarseness / GORD and calf pain / sciatica is arranged

Approach to be taken

A. Data gathering, examination and clinical assessment skills

1. *Define the clinical problem: clarify why the patient has presented today*
   The doctor:
   - makes use of the existing patient information provided prior to the consultation
   - empathises with Mrs SW's comments about needing to make a list because of her 'poor memory'
   - asks the patient to read out the whole list to gauge which problems need urgent attention, which can be dealt with quickly, and which may need attention at a later date. One way of dealing with the list may be to respond with *"OK, that sounds like a reasonable list, all of which need attention. I also need to talk to you about your blood results. Shall we start with that and see how we get on in our ten minutes. If it's OK with you, we'll also make a plan for dealing with those things we may not have time for today."*
   - asks questions to explore how reliable the fasting blood glucose result is and makes arrangements for a glucose tolerance test (GTT)
   - asks open questions to explore what Mrs SW means by menopausal symptoms, which symptoms have the greatest adverse impact on her life and what her expectations of treatment are, thereby eliciting the story of lacking energy and the expectation of treatment to restore her drive
   - asks closed questions to clarify details about her periods, and possible contra-indications to HRT
   - asks about red flags for calf pain (recent swelling or pain, recent long periods of immobility), and hoarse voice (particularly hoarseness that deteriorated over the past month despite proton pump inhibitors)
   - discovers Mrs SW's idea that her lack of energy is due to the menopause, her concern about the risk of DVT with HRT, and her expectation for further information about HRT and a prescription for a lansoprazole

2. *Performs an appropriate physical or mental examination*
   - In this case, an examination is not required.

B. Clinical management skills

3. *Make an appropriate working diagnosis*
   The doctor, based on the history, makes a working diagnosis of:
   - possible disorders of glucose metabolism requiring further investigation (GGT)
   - peri-menopausal symptoms

1

C. Interpersonal skills: know and treat this patient

8. *Achieve rapport*
   The doctor:
   - listens attentively to Mrs SW's recitation of her list without interruption, acknowledging that concern for her ability to remember everything prompted its writing
   - understands her request for information on HRT, a repeat script for a PPI and review of her sciatica; the doctor is sympathetic and outlines his intention to address these issues today and at future appointments
   - displays empathy to her lack of energy and supports her in her attempt to change her lifestyle
   - is non-judgemental about the patient's alcohol intake and congratulates her on the reduction she's made
   - addresses the patient's specific concerns and expectations

9. *Give the patient the opportunity to be involved in significant management decisions*
   The doctor:
   - encourages autonomy and opinions – provides Mrs SW with a brief outline on treatment options and signposts to appropriate resources on HRT management
   - suggests further appointments with appropriate members of the PCT for future review

Debrief

Discuss how the doctor could, if needed, improve his performance. In particular, assess whether the doctor:
- negotiated the patient's list? Was this done in a sensitive manner?
- established and maintained rapport? If so, how?
- addressed Mrs SW's specific expectations? If so, how?
- discussed and signposted to appropriate HRT, including CAM?
- safety netted? If so, how?

If the consultation over-ran, did the doctor:
- spend too much time negotiating the list?
- ask too many questions about all the presenting issues before deciding on the ones to tackle?
- provide detailed information when outlining the main points would have sufficed? Remember that if the actor–patient is unhappy with the amount and detail of information provided, they are briefed to press the issue. In this case, the actor–patient would have been briefed to leave the appointment with a script for her PPI, a follow-up blood test, some information on treatments for the menopause and a strategy for tackling her on-going calf pain/sciatica. An acceptable strategy would be *"let's discuss this further at a follow-up appointment, which you can arrange, at your convenience, with the receptionist."*

Revising data gathering

What questions could the doctor ask to discover the patient's ideas, and expectations? How could the doctor address the patient's concerns and health beliefs?
- Ideas: *"You mention making a list to help you remember? What do you think is making you forgetful? Do you think that feeling low and lacking energy is due to the menopause?"*
- Concerns: *"Your calf pain sounds like on-going sciatica – nerve pain, rather than a DVT. HRT affects the blood and slightly increases the risk of clotting in the veins. HRT should not make your nerve pain worse and your sciatica does not increase your risk of clotting."*
- Expectations: *"Your list allows us to prioritise things so we can tackle them logically. If we can't get through everything, please remind me that I definitely have to discuss your blood results; what do you definitely have to leave with today?"*
- Health beliefs: *"I agree that your symptoms sound like the menopause. How we treat the menopause depends on which symptoms are troubling you most. HRT is probably better for the lack of energy and irregular bleeding, but low mood and hot flushes could be treated with Prozac-type medication, while poor sleep could be treated with regular exercise or valerian. Let me briefly outline each option for you and then give you some written information. How does that sound?"*

Test your theoretical knowledge

For each of the following statements, answer true (T) or false (F).

Regarding hoarseness:
1. Hoarseness due to upper respiratory tract infections resolves spontaneously
2. Hoarseness due to hypothyroidism is likely to resolve with thyroxine treatment
3. Paralysis of the recurrent laryngeal nerve, due to surgical trauma or malignancy, presents with hoarseness
4. If hoarseness persists for more than 6 weeks, refer to a chest physician to exclude oropharyngeal malignancy
5. The effect of inhaled steroids on hoarseness is not dose-related

Relevant literature

www.patient.co.uk/showdoc/40000966/

http://cks.library.nhs.uk/menopause

http://cks.library.nhs.uk/dyspepsia_proven_gord

Case 20 – Dyspepsia

Brief to the doctor

Mr ST, a 45 year old man, has seen you twice in the past 3 months for dyspepsia. One month ago you gave him a prescription for omeprazole 20 mg once daily for 28 days.

Patient summary

Name	ST
Date of birth (Age)	45
Social and family history	Married
Past medical history	3 months ago: GP consultation: "*4months' dyspepsia. No red flags. Smokes 15/day. Alc – 18 units/week. Intermittent diclofenac for back. OTC Gaviscon helps. OE - NAD. Advised – lose weight, stop smoking, no late meals. Stop diclofenac. Gaviscon prn 500mls.*"
	1 month ago: GP consultation: "*Above not helped. Had partic bad episode and OTC ranitidine helped. Back is OK with paracetamol. Still smoking. Has lost some wt – congratulated. Abdo soft. No red flags, so 1m trial PPI. Omeprazole 20mg od ×28. Rev 1m*"
Current medication	Omeprazole 20 mg od Diclofenac 50 mg 1 tds prn for back pain
Investigations BMI BP Tobacco Alcohol	3months ago: 29.3 134/86 15/day 18 units/wk

Tasks for the doctor

In this case, the tasks are to:
1. ascertain Mr ST's response to the PPI trial
2. agree a management plan including lifestyle changes

Brief to the patient – more about the patient

1. Profile:

- Mr ST is 45 years old. He works in the planning department at the local council. He married with 3 teenage children
- His father died 10 years ago of an MI aged 60; mother alive, hypertensive
- Smokes 15/day – he has tried patches and gum in the past, but was never cigarette free for more than 3 weeks
- drinks 18 units/week (wine)

2. He is seeing the doctor today because:

- he has had indigestion for 7 months – the response to omeprazole has been 'miraculous'
- he would like to continue taking the tablets

3. Additional information:

- If the doctor asks specifically:
  - his indigestion symptoms are: upper abdominal pain between meals with some belching. The pain has woken him at night a couple of times in the past. Symptoms worse after big or late meals. No nausea, vomiting, haematemesis, heartburn, dysphagia.
  - he has lost a few pounds
  - he still gets intermittent back pain, but since being told to stop taking diclofenac, he has been able to control this reasonably well with paracetamol and exercises. He thinks this has been a good move, because it has made him do his exercises and watch his posture rather than 'just take a tablet and mask the pain'.
  - he is not concerned he has anything other than plain indigestion and he does not want any investigations
  - he has heard about *H. pylori* and wonders whether he should be tested as this might give him life-long cure
- He enjoys smoking and finds it helps him relax. If the doctor can present him with evidence that he has other risk factors for heart disease, he might be persuaded to give stopping another try.
- He could easily be persuaded to lose weight and change his diet.
- He would like to be more physically active and is open to suggestions on how to lead a more physically active life. He drives to work, dropping the children off at school on the way. They live on the edge of town, just too far to walk into town easily.

Approach to be taken

A. Data gathering, examination and clinical assessment skills

1. *Define the clinical problem: clarify why the patient has presented today*
   The doctor:
   - reads the patient information provided prior to the consultation
   - asks open questions to explore how Mr ST responded to the omeprazole and whether he believes the lifestyle changes he made previously helped: *"How have things been since I saw you last?"*
   - asks closed questions to exclude red flag symptoms signalling the need for referral
   - discovers Mr ST's desire to keep taking omeprazole: *"Have you any ideas about what we should do now?"*
   - clarifies whether Mr ST would like further tests: *"Have you heard about any investigations or tests for this?"*

2. *Performs an appropriate physical or mental examination*
   - In this case, an examination is not required.

B. Clinical management skills

3. *Make an appropriate working diagnosis*
   - The doctor, based on the history, makes a working diagnosis of uninvestigated dyspepsia with no red flags; Mr ST tells you that he is happy with this diagnosis.

4. *Explain the problem to the patient using appropriate language*
   The doctor:
   - having quickly established Mr ST's response to omeprazole, addresses his agenda: wanting to keep taking omeprazole
   - provides some information on the effectiveness of lifestyle changes in the management of dyspepsia

5. *Provide holistic care and use resources effectively*
   The doctor:
   - informs Mr ST about *H. pylori* testing, eradication treatment and success rates and ascertains whether he would like to explore this treatment option
   - discusses the pros and cons of using omeprazole long-term, either continuously or intermittently
   - explores Mr ST's ideas about smoking and the benefits of stopping smoking: *"Have you any thoughts about how smoking might be affecting you?"*
   - identifies other risk factors for CVD: FH, overweight, relative lack of exercise and uses this to try to motivate Mr ST to stop smoking, lose weight and lead a more physically active lifestyle

- congratulates Mr ST for managing his back pain without diclofenac – this is an opportunity to reinforce a message that self-management can be very effective

6. *Prescribe appropriately*
The doctor:
- is aware of national and local guidelines – NICE (2004, revised 2005) *Dyspepsia: management of dyspepsia in adults in primary care*
- negotiates an appropriate treatment option:
  - return to self-management (as per NICE guidelines)
  - intermittent PPI use
  - *H. pylori* testing
- offers smoking cessation advice
- offers advice on diet, weight loss and increased physical activity

7. *Specify the conditions and interval for follow-up*
The doctor:
- signposts Mr ST to information on CVD risk factors
- offers a follow-up appointment either with a doctor or with a nurse to discuss smoking cessation and other lifestyle modifications
- arranges a follow up appointment to review the *H. pylori* test result
- safety nets – informs Mr ST about dyspepsia 'red-flag' symptoms
- confirms understanding – *"Do you have any questions?"*

C. Interpersonal skills: know and treat this patient

8. *Achieve rapport*
The doctor:
- listens actively and explores the patient's health ideas, concerns and expectations
- in particular, explores and clarifies Mr ST's beliefs about medication, smoking and motivation for stopping smoking
- explores ways to motivate the patient to lose weight and to become more physically active
- displays empathy and is non-judgemental about Mr ST's weight and smoking

9. *Give the patient the opportunity to be involved in significant management decisions*
The doctor:
- actively confirms the patient's understanding of the dyspepsia and CVD risk factors: *"Does all this make sense to you?"*
- shares thoughts and involves patient in deciding which management option to select
- encourages autonomy and opinions – provides him with information so he feels able to understand self-management for himself and his family
- supports and congratulates his self-management of his back pain

Debrief

Discuss how the doctor could, if needed, improve his performance. In particular, assess how the doctor:

- negotiated an appropriate management plan for dyspepsia
- discussed CVD risk factors
- tried to motivate Mr ST to stop smoking
- structured the consultation and used the time appropriately

Revising data gathering

What questions could the doctor ask to discover the patient's ideas, concerns, expectations and health beliefs?

- Ideas: "*I understand that you are keen to continue on omeprazole; have you thought about other ways to treat your symptoms?*"
- Concerns: "*You don't seem keen on stopping smoking. Are there any particular reasons?*"
- Expectations: "*It seems that you are not very happy with your current diet; would you like to discuss how it could be improved?*"
- Health beliefs: "*You know that smoking increases your risk of heart disease, but there are other factors as well. Would you like to check over these and see if any apply to you?*"

Test your theoretical knowledge

For each of the following statements, answer true (T) or false (F).

1. A minimum 4 week wash-out period following PPI use is required before testing for *H. pylori* with a breath test
2. Patients over 55 whose symptoms persist despite *H. pylori* eradication or acid suppression treatment should be considered for endoscopy
3. Cognitive behaviour therapy may reduce dyspepsia symptoms in the short-term
4. For patients with persistent symptoms, but no red-flag symptoms, testing for and treating *H. pylori* is more cost effective than further management based on endoscopy
5. The prevalence of *H. pylori* in the UK is around 40%

Relevant literature

Delaney BC, Qume M, Moayyedi P, *et al.* (2008) *Helicobacter pylori* test and treat versus proton pump inhibitor in initial management of dyspepsia in primary care: multicentre randomised controlled trial (MRC-CUBE trial). *BMJ*, **336:** 651–654.

NICE (2004, revised 2005) *Dyspepsia: management of dyspepsia in adults in primary care* (CG17): http://guidance.nice.org.uk/CG17).

Preparing for the MRCGP Clinical Skills Assessment (CSA)

In this section, we shall discuss:
- how to use the practice cases, including
  - the 'patient'
  - the 'doctor'
  - the 'examiner'
  - the usefulness of these scenarios for group CSA practice
- information about the CSA, including:
  - the structure of the CSA
  - what happens on the exam day
  - the marking of the CSA
  - preparing for the CSA

How to use the practice cases

The following practice cases will help GP trainees prepare for Clinical Skills Assessment (CSA). They are written for use in a study group, ideally consisting of three trainees.

Please note that some of the practice cases were originally published in *GP*, and are reproduced here with permission (www.gponline.com).

The 'patient'
The trainee playing the 'patient' should read the 'brief to the patient' section to enable her to understand the expectations of the patient so she can then answer the doctor's questions. If an examination is expected, the patient is briefed about the findings and may have to make up a card containing the relevant information prior to starting the consultation. If the patient brief does not contain this information, for example a BP reading, and the doctor wishes to examine the patient, the patient should allow the examination to actually occur. Performing irrelevant or unjustified examinations eats into the consultation time. If the 'doctor' asks to perform intimate examinations not contained within the patient brief, the patient should decline.

The 'doctor'
The 'doctor' should read the 'patient medical record' section at the start of the consultation because it contains a summary of the patient's relevant details. A recent test result, such as a fasting glucose result, may be provided. Sometimes, a copy of the last patient consultation is given. The background information often provides a clue about today's consultation or gives important data relevant to today's management decisions.

The 'examiner'

Ideally, the third trainee playing the 'examiner' should enter the consulting room with the patient and sit unobtrusively where the 'doctor' cannot see him. The examiner should mark the case using the 'marking guide' by ticking against the positive or negative indicators as the consultation unfolds. At the end of the consultation, the examiner should also make a global judgement of whether the 'doctor', based on this consultation, is fit for independent practice. The 'examiner' times the case, sounding an alarm when the ten minutes are up.

The usefulness of these scenarios for group CSA practice

The CSA tests the candidate's ability to gather and assess medical information, make structured, evidence-based and flexible decisions and communicate with patients in a way that moves the consultation forward in an ethical and responsible manner. The candidate passes if he or she is able to ask the patient the right questions, at the right time, in the right way, perform the right examination correctly and communicate effectively, all within ten minutes. The marking grid in each practice case for CSA study groups provides the model for an ordered, step-wise approach to data gathering, management and communication. However, the group debrief, using the debrief prompts at the end of each case, is essential to review the actual performance. The group feedback informs the doctor about his current knowledge and communication skills and advises him on how he can improve his performance for success in the CSA.

Information about the CSA

The structure of the CSA

The CSA is one of the three components of the MRCGP assessment. It is designed to test a doctor's ability to ***integrate*** and ***apply*** clinical, professional, communication and practical skills appropriate for general practice, "to produce a consultation that is meaningful to both patient and doctor and which moves the patient forward towards a justifiable management of their presenting problem" (Hawthorne, 2007).

What happens on exam day

- On the day of the examination, at the examination venue, each candidate is given a consulting room.
- The candidate is briefed to treat the examination session as if he is a locum doctor.
- He is to interact with the patient and not the examiner, who will remain a silent observer.
- The candidate's surgery has thirteen booked patients who enter his consulting room when the buzzer sounds.
- At the end of 10 minutes, the buzzer sounds to signal the departure of the patient.
- There is a two minute gap between consultations.
- Twelve patients are true examination cases on which the candidate is assessed. One is a 'trial station' in which new clinical scenarios are trialled. The candidate will not know which is the trial case.
- There will be a short break in the middle of surgery.

The marking of CSA
The patients, played by trained actors, will move from room to room, together with the examiner for that case. Each examiner will mark the same case all day, thus providing standardised marking.

Each case is marked in three domains, and all have equal weighting.
- *Data gathering, examination and clinical assessment skills*: the ability to take a targeted history and perform a focused physical examination. Candidates are expected to be knowledgeable and skilful in their examination techniques and in the appropriate use of medical instruments. Marks are awarded for the fluency with which procedures are performed.
- *Clinical management skills*: in line with current accepted British general practice.
- *Interpersonal skills:* the candidate shows an ability to engage patients in the consultation, using recognised interpersonal skills, such as enquiring about the patient's health beliefs and incorporating these into the explanation given to the patient. Some cases also assess the candidate's ability to value patients' contributions, and to respect their autonomy and decision-making.

The pass mark is set as the standard required to practise independently as a licensed GP. The candidate is then given an overall grade, namely a Clear Pass, Marginal Pass, Marginal Fail or Clear Fail.

In very simple terms, data-gathering is about ***how*** you get to the 'nub' of the presenting problem; clinical management is about ***what*** you do to move the problem forward; and interpersonal skills is about ***how*** you go about doing it.

Each case is written to focus on a particular 'nub'. The marking schedule, using positive and negative indicators of practice, reflects this nub. Please refer to video cases 8 to 13 for examples of the marking schedule.

Preparing for CSA
Do the job. The CSA cases are all written by GPs active in the UK National Health Service and reflect real-life presentations. Therefore, candidates with some experience in NHS general practice should not have difficulty with the exam. The RCGP recommends that candidates first complete at least 6 months of UK NHS GP practice before sitting the exam.

Read the website. Candidates are advised to read the Curriculum Statements from the RCGP website. Each curriculum statement has a section on common and important conditions and cases are quite likely to be based on one of these.

Analyse your consultations. Candidates are advised to video their own consultations, watch them with a colleague, and analyse them for the clinical approach and interpersonal skills displayed. Alternatively, candidates may work in small groups, practising cases such as the ones contained in this section of the book.

Practise clinical examinations. Candidates are advised to practise the focused examinations that are most likely to be tested, such as assessment of a limb, chest or abdomen. Some examinations, such as intimate examinations on a role player, or examinations that might cause discomfort if repeated, are less likely to be tested. Candidates are advised to be familiar and confident with medical equipment, such as otoscopes.

Interpret data. Candidates are advised to become familiar with the letters GPs receive from secondary care, and test results such as ECGs, spirometry, blood tests, urinalysis, skin scrapings and swabs. Candidates need to ensure that they can interpret results correctly and explain them to a patient.

The practice CSA cases in this section of the book include cases that require candidates to practise physical examination and interpret test results.

Additional reading

Malik S (2006) An OSCE actress. *BMJ Career Focus,* **332**: 110.

Ms Malik describes her experience as an OCSE actress, how she was briefed to play the case, and what examiners asked of her regarding the candidates. She also gives her tips on how candidates should prepare:

> "I would suggest that if you can sense the acting patient is not happy with the situation then you should ask: *"Is there anything I've said that is confusing or not clear or that you want explained again?"* Another tip is to have a mental checklist of questions prepared and if you find yourself in an awkward situation, go back to where you left off in the list."

Relevant literature

Hawthorne K (2007) Introduction to the cases in the Clinical Skills Assessment. RCGP website: www.rcgp-curriculum.org.uk/nmrgcp/csa/csa_cases.aspx

Simpson RG (2007) Preparing for practice: nMRCGP and the Clinical Skills Assessment. *Update,* **75**: 36–37.

Royal College of General Practitioners nMRCGP website: www.rcgp-curriculum.org.uk/examinations_and_assessment.aspx, particularly:
- www.rcgp-curriculum.org.uk/PDF/curr_1_Curriculum_Statement_Being_a_GP.pdf for the GP curriculum – the core statement
- www.rcgp.org.uk/pdf/curriculum_Guide_for_Learners_and_Teachers.pdf for in-depth reading of learning outcomes for general practice

Practice case 1 – Medication request for daughter

Brief to the patient

- You are Katie Perret, a 29 year old mum. You present today without your children to obtain a prescription for 2½ year old Anne and to ask for advice about 5 year old Olivia's night terrors.
- When you consulted with Anne ten days ago, the doctor agreed with you that Anne's persistent night-time cough and her occasional wheeze may be caused by asthma. She advised you to try a blue salbutamol inhaler. Anne used the inhaler and the face mask without difficulty. It has made some difference but she is not completely better.
- Anne has used the inhaler 2–3 times per day. Thirty minutes after using the inhaler, her cough recurs. You are not sure if the blue inhaler alone is adequate medication. You have been asthmatic since childhood and based on your experience, you feel Anne needs a brown steroid inhaler.
- You are concerned about the night-time cough. It still disturbs Olivia who has to wake up for school the next morning. You are also worried about Olivia's night terrors. Is the poor sleep making the night terrors worse? Is there anything you could do to help Olivia with her night terrors?
- Olivia has had night terrors from the age of 3. The health visitor advised a good night routine for Olivia, but despite this she tends to get one at least once a week. If questioned, it usually happens two hours after she falls asleep. She bolts upright in bed, screams like mad, looks ashen, cries inconsolably and never remembers it in the morning. It is difficult to rouse her in the middle of a terror.
- You would like to get a prescription for a brown steroid inhaler for Anne and some advice for Olivia. You didn't think Anne needed to be re-examined today. She is usually fine during the day and at the last consultation, the doctor did not detect anything untoward on examination. You really don't think it is worth coming back with the children for medication to be issued. If you are asked to return before a prescription is issued, you want to know what the examination will add to the consultation.

Patient medical record for the doctor

Name   Anne Perret (2½ years old)

Consultation note by GP (ten days ago)
'Mum had asthma from age 5. Anne occasionally has cough at night (after 9pm) and over last few nights, mum noticed wheeze. Kept sister (school age) awake. Tried steam

This practice case originally appeared in *GP* and is reproduced here in an amended form with permission (see **www.gponline.com**)

inhalation / propping up head of bed, but did not help. Frustrated as presented many times with cough and told it is a self-limiting viral illness. O/E: chest sounds normal; no wheeze. Tearing up surgery, healthy looking. Plan: try salbutamol inhaler and review if needed.'

Marking guide for the assessor

Generic indicators for targeted assessment domains	Descriptors – positive and negative
A. Data gathering, technical and assessment skills: • Gathering of data for clinical judgement, choice of examination, investigations and their interpretations. • Demonstrating proficiency in performing physical examinations and using diagnostic and therapeutic instruments.	Positive indicators: • Reads the previous consultation prior to the patient's presentation. • Asks open questions to clarify the nature of the problem followed by closed questions to understand exactly what mum is requesting today. • The doctor systematically excludes red flags (intercurrent illness; severe asthma) that may signal the need for in-person review. • Comes to an understanding of how Anne's night-time cough exacerbates Olivia's night terrors and the impact on the family. • Elicits mum's concerns about Anne's 'partially treated asthma' and her expectations of a prescription. Negative indicators: • The doctor fails to respond to mum's cues about 'disturbed sleep'. By not establishing the link between disturbed sleep and Olivia's worsening night terrors, the doctor does not provide holistic family care.

B. Clinical management skills • Recognition and management of common medical conditions in primary care. Demonstrates flexible and structured approach to decision-making. • Demonstrating ability to deal with multiple complaints and co-morbidity and to promote a shared approach to managing problems.	Positive indicators: • Makes a clinically sound working diagnosis on the basis of probability. Either offers a test for asthma or initiates Step 2 asthma treatment on a trial basis. • The explanation about interrupted sleep aggravating night terrors is logical and incorporates the patient's beliefs. • Advises about the treatment of night terrors. • Outlines when follow-up or review is needed (safety-nets). If referral to the asthma nurse is offered, mum is given sufficient information to make a decision. Negative indicators: • Fails to prescribe safely, or in line with current best practice, or fails to justify why a prescription is given or withheld. • Fails to check the patient's understanding of the medication and/or her ability to use the medication appropriately. • Fails to formulate a management plan for night terrors or fails to advise why this needs to be addressed in a separate consultation.
C. Interpersonal skills • Use of recognised communication techniques that enhance understanding of a patient's illness and promote a shared approach to managing problems. • Practising ethically with respect for equality and diversity in line with accepted codes of professional conduct.	Positive indicators: • Listens attentively and empathises with adverse effect of nocturnal cough on the family. • Is non-judgemental about mum's ideas; refrains from retorting, 'So you think a steroid inhaler is needed. At which medical school did you train?' • Encourages mum's opinions and autonomy but maintains primary duty of care to the children. Negative indicators: • The doctor interrupts unnecessarily and breaks the flow of conversation. • The doctor's manner discourages questioning or the sharing of opinions. • The patient is not offered options regarding treatment or follow-up.

Group debrief

Discuss how the doctor could, if needed, improve his or her performance.

In particular, assess whether the doctor 'showed poor time management':
- How long did the doctor take to obtain the history? Was questioning efficient, appropriately selective or needlessly repetitive?
- Was the second half of the consultation (clinical management, explaining and follow-up arrangements) rushed?
- Were the relevant psychosocial factors covered?

In the group, discuss whether the doctor developed an adequate management plan:
- What was the management plan? Was it appropriate to the level of risk?
- Were the possible risks and benefits of different management approaches, including prescribing, clearly identified and discussed?

Relevant literature

van Dorp F. (2008) Consultations with children. *InnovAiT*, **1 (1):** 54–61.

Driver H.S. & Shapiro C.M. (1993) ABC of sleep disorders. Parasomnias. *BMJ*, **306:** 921 doi:10.1136/bmj.306.6882.921

Practice case 2 – Alcohol detoxification

Brief to the patient

- You are Martin Rice, a 41 year old unmarried municipal gardener. You are brought in today by your work colleague Jim, who on visiting your flat, found you wrapped in a duvet and throwing up. You smell of alcohol.
- You present as an emergency. Jim was concerned that you hadn't reported to work after a week of sick leave, which you were given by the consultant psychiatrist last week. The psychiatrist thought your feelings of panic were due to your medication (venlafaxine) being dropped from 75 mg to 37.5 mg, so he increased it back to 75mg once daily and also prescribed some diazepam. You took all the diazepam in the first two days, but because you continued to feel panicky, you drank alcohol.
- Jim confirms that you drank 6 litres of vodka over the week. He found the empty bottles in your room. Unless asked, Jim sits quietly in the room and lets you speak.
- You are adamant that you usually drink hardly any alcohol. You binged over the last six days to self-medicate the anxiety. The medication changes did not touch the anxiety and you 'want help'.
- If asked, you admit to feeling very agitated and your legs feel restless. You have not been sweating excessively. You say you do not have a tremor; you have not had any hallucinations or periods of confusion. You have not been using recreational drugs.
- If questioned about your past history, you have been on venlafaxine for two years to treat depression. About 12 months ago you were admitted to hospital for a brief period when you experienced a similar reaction when your medication was reduced. You barely remember the details, only that the nurses were very rude and you eventually self-discharged because they were not helping you.
- You want further time off work to allow the venlafaxine to work. You want tablets stronger than the diazepam to help your anxiety. If advised that it is not safe for you to go home alone, you say you can go to your mother's house in Stafford. You offer the GP your mother's mobile number. You prefer not to be hospitalised.
- You appear very agitated with fidgety legs and hands throughout the consultation.

Patient medical record for the doctor

Name	Martin Rice (41 years)
Past medical history	Depression (moderate to severe) 2009 Left scaphoid fracture 2005
Current medication	Venlafaxine 37.5 mg once daily

This practice case originally appeared in *GP* and is reproduced here in an amended form with permission (see **www.gponline.com**)

Consultation by patient's usual GP (ten days ago)

'Two weeks ago reduced venlafaxine to 37.5 mg and starting to feel he is in a downward spiral, mood dropped, difficulty focusing at work. Started drinking 2 days ago and turned up to work drunk yesterday. No withdrawals or cravings. No thoughts of DSH. Lives alone. Gets nightmares and struggles to stay asleep. Plan: patient keen to get back to work. Will increase meds back to 75 mg. Advised to throw alcohol away. I will write to psychiatrist to request review appointment brought forward to this week.'

Marking guide for the assessor

Generic indicators for targeted assessment domains	Descriptors – positive and negative
A. Data gathering, technical and assessment skills: • Gathering of data for clinical judgement, choice of examination, investigations and their interpretations. • Demonstrating proficiency in performing physical examinations and using diagnostic and therapeutic instruments.	Positive indicators: • Asks selective questions, tailored to establishing what has triggered the patient's anxiety and restlessness. • Enquires about the medication, possible side effects, dosing regime and compliance. Takes a comprehensive alcohol and drug history. • Enquires about red flags, such as delirium tremens (DTs), deliberate self-harm (DSH) and risk to others from the patient's driving and occupation. Negative indicators: • Questioning and examination is not sufficiently selective. Most questions should address the alcohol issue so you can safely manage the patient's withdrawal symptoms. • The patient's use of diazepam or other drugs and the co-existence of physical or psychiatric illness are not explored. • Details of the patient's support network are not obtained.

B. Clinical management skills	Positive indicators:
• Recognition and management of common medical conditions in primary care. Demonstrates flexible and structured approach to decision-making. • Demonstrating ability to deal with multiple complaints and co-morbidity and to promote a shared approach to managing problems.	• Doctors discuss what they feel is the safest course of action and explain their reasoning. • Management options, including possible hospital admission or management in the community, are openly discussed. • Management is appropriate to the patient's level of risk, the doctor's experience, and the ability to enlist the help of support networks and agencies. • Doctors advise appropriately on work and driving. Negative indicators: • Doctors fail to manage safely or in line with current best practice. • Follow-up arrangements are inadequate.
C. Interpersonal skills	Positive indicators:
• Use of recognised communication techniques that enhance understanding of a patient's illness and promote a shared approach to managing problems. • Practising ethically with respect for equality and diversity in line with accepted codes of professional conduct.	• Doctors display a good mix of empathy and direction. • They communicate effectively with the patient, not his colleague. • Doctors obtain the patient's permission to discuss issues in front of the colleague or with his mother by telephone. • They develop a shared management plan, stressing what is safe management for the patient and others around him (work colleagues / road users) who could be harmed. Negative indicators: • The doctor assumes the patient cannot provide a history and communicates with the work colleague. • The doctor's non-verbal communication and language is doctor-centred, potentially creating a parent–child dynamic. • The doctor appears judgemental about the use of alcohol.

Group debrief

- What questioning or examining enabled the doctor to differentiate between acute alcohol withdrawal, DTs or serotonin discontinuation syndrome? Was the line of questioning methodical or erratic? Was the history taking tailored or did the doctor ask a battery of non-selective, rote psychiatric questions?
- Did the doctor recognise significant findings: no support at home, co-existing depression, previous self-discharge possibly from in-patient detoxification. How did the doctor use this information to negotiate a safe management plan?
- The most common reason for failure in the CSA is that the doctor does not develop a management plan (including prescribing and referral) reflecting knowledge of current best practice. Did the doctor manage this patient in line with current UK best practice?
- Doctors with good interpersonal skills actively listen, appear to really want to know the patient's answers, and skilfully weave the patient's ideas, concerns and expectations into their management plan. Assess whether this consultation was doctor- or patient-centred and suggest how it could safely be made more patient-centred.

Relevant literature

NICE Clinical Guideline (June 2010) Alcohol-use disorders: physical complications. http://guidance.nice.org.uk/CG100

Parker A.J., Marshall E.J. & Ball D.M. (2008) Diagnosis and management of alcohol use disorders. *BMJ*, **336:** 496–501.

Scottish Intercollegiate Guidelines Network (SIGN) (2003) The management of harmful drinking and alcohol dependence in primary care.

Practice case 3 – Paediatric conjunctivitis

Brief to the patient

- You are Paula Hayden, a 25 year old mum. You called the practice to check if your baby's eye swab result has arrived.
- The receptionist informed you that the results are available but she cannot pass them to you. She placed your name in the duty doctor's clinic for him or her to call you back.
- Your baby, Tom, developed sticky eyes when he was five days old. Your GP took a swab and prescribed chloramphenicol eye ointment which you have been using for four days.
- Tom still has sticky eyes but does not seem to be unwell. This morning you noticed a slight streak of blood on his eyelid. You are not sure if this is from scratching, perhaps because of ongoing discomfort. You wanted to check if the 'right' antibiotic was prescribed, hence you called for the swab result.
- You are concerned about Chlamydia eye infection. Your husband had a one-night stand a few months ago. He went to the GUM clinic for treatment and you took antibiotics on their advice. You have read on the internet that Chlamydia can cause conjunctivitis.
- You and your husband have discussed his infidelity. You have forgiven him and believe that he has been faithful since. However, you are concerned about Tom and angry that he is 'suffering' from an eye infection.
- If questioned, Tom was born by vaginal delivery five days after your due date. There were no problems during your pregnancy and labour. His baby check prior to discharge was fine. He feeds well and except for his eye infection, you have no concerns.
- You are happy to bring Tom for a doctor's appointment later today. You plan to travel to your mum's house in North Wales early tomorrow morning. You will be on holiday for two weeks. You would prefer to get any 'new' antibiotics from your GP before you leave. You are not keen to take your baby to the GUM clinic.

Patient medical record for the doctor

Name   Tom Hayden (9 days old)

Note by receptionist (today)
Mum (Paula) called for eye swab result. Advised that duty doctor will call her later on 07744 226688. Telephone appointment made.

Specimen   Eye swab (today)

Chlamydia PCR *C. trachomatis* DNA detected (CDR). Patient and partner STD screening available at GUM. Patients may telephone directly for an appointment on 0745 910 3355.

Consultation note by GP (four days ago)

'Developed bilateral sticky eyes 5 days ago. Parents concerned about Chlamydia – openly discussed. Swab taken. Chloramphenicol prescribed.'

Marking guide for the assessor

Generic indicators for targeted assessment domains	Descriptors – positive and negative
A. Data gathering, technical and assessment skills: • Gathering of data for clinical judgement, choice of examination, investigations and their interpretations. • Demonstrating proficiency in performing physical examinations and using diagnostic and therapeutic instruments.	Positive indicators: • Establishes the identity of the caller and patient. • Asks open questions to clarify the nature of the problem followed by closed questions to understand exactly what the mum is requesting today. • The doctor systematically excludes red flags signalling the need for in-person review or referral. This is important; the difficulty with telephone triage is the ability to make management decisions in the absence of visual cues. Negative indicators: • It would be difficult to do a telephone consultation, especially one on a sensitive topic, without first establishing identity and rapport. • The doctor fails to read and understand the medical information provided prior to phoning. • The doctor fails to elicit the patient's concerns about Chlamydia before discussing the swab results. • The doctor fails to elicit the patient's expectation for new antibiotics.

B. Clinical management skills	Positive indicators:
• Recognition and management of common medical conditions in primary care. Demonstrates flexible and structured approach to decision-making. • Demonstrating ability to deal with multiple complaints and co-morbidity and to promote a shared approach to managing problems.	• Treats Chlamydia eye infection in line with current guidance: erythromycin 50 mg/kg/day in 4 divided doses. Topical treatment is not required. • Gives information about Chlamydia eye infection and sexual health in digestable chunks. The patient's understanding is checked at each step. • Management addresses Mrs Hayden's concerns and expectations. • Outlines when follow-up or review is needed (safety-nets). • Summarises well and ends with 'Are you happy with these arrangements?'
	Negative indicators:
	• Doctors fail to prescribe safely or in line with current best practice. • Chlamydia and marital issues are not explored holistically. • Follow-up arrangements are inadequately discussed.
C. Interpersonal skills	Positive indicators:
• Use of recognised communication techniques that enhance understanding of a patient's illness and promote a shared approach to managing problems. • Practising ethically with respect for equality and diversity in line with accepted codes of professional conduct.	• Listens attentively to Mrs Hayden's request for advice regarding Tom's ongoing eye symptoms. • Questions in a systematic manner but takes care not to 'interrogate' the patient. • Explores her request for advice from the duty doctor today and refrains from making comments such as 'Why couldn't you wait for your GP to call you?'
	Negative indicators:
	• The doctor interrupts unnecessarily and breaks the flow of conversation. • The doctor lacks sensitivity in his or her queries regarding Chlamydia and marital issues. • The doctor fails to encourage autonomy and opinions. The patient is not offered options regarding treatment or follow-up.

Group debrief

Discuss how the doctor could, if needed, improve his or her performance. In particular, assess whether the doctor:

- established rapport on the telephone? If so, how?
- established Mrs Hayden's reasons for calling, her specific concerns and expectations? If so, how?
- summarised and checked understanding?

A common reason for failure in the CSA is that the doctor 'does not identify the patient's agenda, health beliefs and preferences or does not make use of verbal and non-verbal cues'. In the group, discuss what specific questions the doctor could ask to discover the patient's ideas, concerns, expectations and health beliefs? Do these questions blend into the conversation? Which questions sound out-of-place, as if asked by rote? If the questions sound clunky, how would you rephrase them?

Relevant literature

For guidance on management see: www.bmj.com/cgi/reprint/2/6142/961-a

For guidance on telephone consultations, see
Car J. & Sheikh A. (2003) Telephone consultations. *BMJ*, **326:** 966–969; doi:10.1136/bmj.326.7396.966. Box 2 on page 968 is useful.

Practice case 4 – Temporary resident requests medication

Brief to the patient

- You are Mariam Aziz, a 71 year old pensioner. Today you travelled from Glasgow to visit your son and his family.
- You present as an emergency because you forgot to pack your blood pressure medication.
- Your son called your Glasgow practice and spoke to the receptionist who read out the list of medication on your repeat script, namely bendroflumethiazide 2.5 mg once daily, atenolol 50 mg once daily, aspirin 75 mg once daily, and diazepam 2 mg at night.
- Your son accompanies you into the consultation to introduce you to his GP and because he has the list of medication.
- You speak good English. If asked, you don't mind your son coming in with you. However, if probed about your medical issues, you become uncomfortable discussing these in your son's presence and would prefer that the doctor ask him to leave the room.
- When you give the doctor the list of medication, you mention that a week ago, the hospital heart doctor recently added a tablet because the heart was 'getting weaker'. You are unable to remember the tablet's name. Your feet are not swollen and your pulse today is 64 bpm and regular.
- If questioned about the diazepam in front of your son, you are reluctant to discuss the issue. If on your own, you discuss your grief at your husband's death two years ago, your subsequent depression and insomnia. You stopped the anti-depressants but when you tried stopping the diazepam, you felt anxious and couldn't sleep. The psychiatrist advised that you continue with a small dose of diazepam at night. You want the diazepam prescribed and become upset and challenge the doctor if he or she seems reluctant to prescribe it.
- You are happy for the doctor to call your GP and issue a script later.
- You come across as a quiet, unassuming woman but when asked, you have opinions on what you want.
- You are also slightly hard of hearing and if the doctor speaks too quietly (or too rapidly), you ask him or her to repeat the information.

Patient medical record for the doctor

Name Mariam Aziz (71 years)

Past medical history Not known – patient is a temporary resident

---

This practice case originally appeared in *GP* and is reproduced here in an amended form with permission (see **www.gponline.com**)

Marking guide for the assessor

Generic indicators for targeted assessment domains	Descriptors – positive and negative
A. Data gathering, technical and assessment skills: • Gathering of data for clinical judgement, choice of examination, investigations and their interpretations. • Demonstrating proficiency in performing physical examinations and using diagnostic and therapeutic instruments.	Positive indicators: • Establishes rapport with Mrs Aziz and is mindful of discussing her medical issues in front of her son. • Asks open questions (to explore the medication request) followed by closed questions to clarify how the list was compiled and whether the repeat script includes the 'new' tablet. • Enquires about the medication, possible side effects, dosing regime and compliance. • Excludes red flags, such as heart failure or arrhythmias. Negative indicators: • Questioning is not sufficiently detailed. Most questions should address a medication review to enable safe prescribing. • The patient's use of diazepam is not explored. • If a physical examination is undertaken, examination skills are neither sufficiently selective nor fluent.

B. Clinical management skills	Positive indicators:
• Recognition and management of common medical conditions in primary care. Demonstrates flexible and structured approach to decision-making. • Demonstrating ability to deal with multiple complaints and co-morbidity and to promote a shared approach to managing problems.	• Doctors discuss what they feel is the safest course of action and explain their reasoning. • Management options, including writing a script following a telephone call to the patient's GP, are openly discussed and offered to the patient. • Management is appropriate to the patient's level of risk. If new medication is to be prescribed, the need for follow-up is discussed. Negative indicators: • Doctors fail to prescribe safely or in line with current best practice. • Follow-up arrangements are inadequately discussed.
C. Interpersonal skills	Positive indicators:
• Use of recognised communication techniques that enhance understanding of a patient's illness and promote a shared approach to managing problems. • Practising ethically with respect for equality and diversity in line with accepted codes of professional conduct.	• Doctors display rapport-building skills; they communicate effectively with the patient, not her son, using appropriate language and volume. • Doctors identify the patient's embarrassment at discussing her medical details in front of her son and respond appropriately. • They develop a <u>shared</u> management plan, which incorporates the patient's specific concerns about diazepam withdrawal. Negative indicators: • The doctor assumes the patient cannot speak English and communicates with her son. • The language is not pitched at the right level for this patient. • The doctor repeatedly speaks too softly or too loudly. • The doctor appears judgemental about the use of diazepam.

Group debrief

- Assess the doctor's verbal and non-verbal response to the patient and her son. Were assumptions made about the patient based on her ethnic or cultural background?
- Was the patient's medical confidence preserved?
- Was the doctor respectful?
- Did the doctor seem genuinely interested in helping the patient obtain her medication and in prescribing safely?
- Was the patient given the opportunity and time to answer questions?
- Was there a shared management plan that incorporated the patient's concerns and expectations?
- A common reason for failure in the CSA is that the doctor 'does not identify the patient's agenda, health beliefs and preferences or does not make use of verbal and non-verbal cues'. Did the doctor detect and respond to the patient becoming uncomfortable with detailed questioning in her son's presence?
- Another common reason for failure is that the doctor 'does not recognise the challenge' (e.g. the patient's problem or ethical dilemma). Evaluate whether the doctor was mindful of the recent cardiology recommendation and checked if this had been added to the patient's repeat medication. Evaluate whether the patient's medical confidence was protected throughout the consultation.

Relevant literature

For guidance on undertaking medication reviews, see
www.npc.nhs.uk/review_medicines/intro/

Practice case 5 – Insomnia

Brief to the patient

- You are Rodney Heron, a 33 year old married telecommunications engineer. You present today because you had one of the worst night's sleep earlier this week and want advice on insomnia.
- On Sunday you went to bed at 11 pm, your usual time. You finally dozed off at 3 am. After 3–4 hours of sleep, you felt incredibly tired at work. This is becoming an increasingly common occurrence. You worry about not being able to fall asleep, waking up unrefreshed and feeling tired at work. You haven't made any errors at work but you double-check things now so jobs take longer.
- If asked, the problem started insidiously, about two years ago. Nothing happened to trigger the problem; it just developed. You have poor sleep about three or four nights out of seven. You have difficulty getting off to sleep, but once asleep you are fine. You wake up once to use the toilet, but fall asleep within minutes of returning to bed. You do not have any physical discomforts that wake you.
- You reduced your caffeine intake, you exercise early each evening and you keep the bedroom cool and dark.
- You think your mattress may be too hard (you slept better on holiday 2 weeks ago) but purchasing a new mattress would strain your budget at present. You are not keen on medication; colleagues have warned you how addictive sleeping tablets can be. You want some information so that you can decide if it is safe to try Nytol.
- If asked, you are not depressed; your mood is normal. Your wife has not told you that you have odd or loud breathing sounds or agitated movements when you sleep.
- Two years ago, after your dad had a heart attack, you lost 2 stone, gave up smoking and restricted your alcohol intake to 2 bottles of wine over weekends. It is important to you to maintain a healthy lifestyle. You are not obese and your collar size is 15.
- You want to understand why your sleeping has been affected. If the doctor suggests medication, you want to know the risk of addiction. If asked, you are open to alternative treatments; perhaps these are safer than prescription tablets.

Patient medical record for the doctor

Name	Rodney Heron (33 years)
Past medical history	Surgery for bilateral bunions 2008 Obesity due to excess calories 2006
Current medication	None

This practice case originally appeared in *GP* and is reproduced here in an amended form with permission (see www.gponline.com)

Marking guide for the assessor

Generic indicators for targeted assessment domains	Descriptors – positive and negative
A. Data gathering, technical and assessment skills: • Gathering of data for clinical judgement, choice of examination, investigations and their interpretations. • Demonstrating proficiency in performing physical examinations and using diagnostic and therapeutic instruments.	Positive indicators: • Asks open questions about the sleeping problem, daytime sleepiness/napping and factors interfering with sleep. • Asks closed questions to clarify details and exclude secondary causes of insomnia: depression, alcohol, drugs, sleep apnoea and parasomnias. • Elicits how the problem affects the patient, his family and his work. • Discovers his health beliefs and expectations. Negative indicators: • Questioning and examination is not sufficiently selective. Does not obtain sufficient information to support a diagnosis of primary insomnia. • Failure to work through a diagnostic sieve and actively exclude secondary causes of insomnia. • Details of the patient's agenda and health beliefs are not obtained or believed. The doctor persists in asking about hidden agendas such as depression despite the patient not reporting symptoms of a mood disorder.

B. Clinical management skills • Recognition and management of common medical conditions in primary care. Demonstrates flexible and structured approach to decision-making. • Demonstrating ability to deal with multiple complaints and co-morbidity and to promote a shared approach to managing problems.	Positive indicators: • Doctors discuss what they feel the problem is (primary insomnia) and explain their reasoning, using the patient's ideas and beliefs. • Management options, including 'sleep hygiene', restriction of time in bed, drugs, alternative remedies, are openly discussed. • Management addresses the patient's concerns and expectations. • Doctors advise appropriately on work, including the possible impact of a two-week sleep restriction programme on driving. Negative indicators: • Doctors fail to explain the diagnosis or treatment options in jargon-free language. • The evidence base for various treatments is not provided in a simple format. • The patient is not given sufficient information to make informed decisions. • Follow-up arrangements are inadequate.
C. Interpersonal skills • Use of recognised communication techniques that enhance understanding of a patient's illness and promote a shared approach to managing problems. • Practising ethically with respect for equality and diversity in line with accepted codes of professional conduct.	Positive indicators: • Doctors listen attentively and summarise appropriately. • They communicate effectively using the patient's ideas and beliefs. • Doctors involve the patient in decisions, offering choices and encouraging autonomy. Negative indicators: • The doctor assumes the patient wants medication; the patient's understanding of the available options is not explored. • The doctor's repeated questions on depression or drugs create the impression that he or she strongly suspects a hidden agenda. • The doctor is unable to discuss the evidence base in a simple and meaningful way.

Group debrief

- Did the doctor ask sufficient questions in sufficient detail to make a diagnosis of primary insomnia? Did the history-taking feel like an interrogation or a conversation? Did the doctor use rote questions that interrupted the flow of the conversation?
- Did the doctor provide management options? Did he or she discuss the pros and cons of 'sleep hygiene', restriction of time in bed, over the counter medications (sedating antihistamines, melatonin, valerian), hypnotic drugs or sedating antidepressants or antipsychotics?
- Some cases in the CSA appear simple. Have the confidence to explore hidden agendas and if they are not present (in this case, by establishing the patient is not depressed or requesting specific medication for illicit purposes), move on. Have the courage to take the patient at face value, as you would in your consulting room.
- This case tests whether the doctor can discuss management options meaningfully with the patient. Is the doctor comfortable with discussing the evidence base? Is the doctor prepared to talk about complementary medicine? This case was not written to check for 'hidden agendas' so beware of second-guessing the examiner. Treat what is in front of you.

Relevant literature

Falloon K. *et al.* (2011) The assessment and management of insomnia in primary care. *BMJ*, **342:** d2899.

Practice case 6 – Stress at work

Brief to the patient

- You are Amanda Shaw, a 51 year old hospital nurse, divorced and living alone.
- You have come to see the doctor today as an emergency on the advice of your friend, with whom you are spending a few days. Your friend is extremely worried about your low mood.
- You feel 'stressed at work' mainly because the ward manager is piling on loads of work in preparation for the Health Care Commission (HCC) visit in 2 weeks. She takes credit for your ideas, expects you to carry a clinical and administrative workload and undermines you in front of team members. You feel unable to talk to her because she is abrasive and does not listen.
- If asked specifically, you admit to having a low mood for two months, increasing irritability, crying easily, a loss of confidence, difficulty sleeping and 'panic', moments when you feel very anxious. You are not suicidal. You have not suffered from depression before.
- If questioned in detail, you admit to stopping your HRT 3 months ago after developing vaginal bleeding. Your hysteroscopy was 'horrible' and you don't want to restart HRT. Occasionally (once per fortnight), you are woken up by hot flushes.
- You think you have 'work stress' and difficulty dealing with it because of your menopausal symptoms.
- You want a sick note for 3 weeks, until after the HCC visit, so you can stay with your friend and 'get your head around issues'.
- You are worried that your manager and team will think you are a 'shirker' if you request annual leave but you are also concerned that your lack of concentration will result in errors at work which will land you in even bigger trouble with the RCN.
- You do not want 'pills' or 'referrals'. You feel the problem lies with your manager and you don't need 'fixing'.
- You cry intermittently throughout this consultation.

Patient medical record for the doctor

Name   Amanda Shaw (51 years)

Past medical history   Not known – patient is a temporary resident

This practice case originally appeared in *GP* and is reproduced here in an amended form with permission (see **www.gponline.com**)

Marking guide for the assessor

Generic indicators for targeted assessment domains	Descriptors – positive and negative
A. Data gathering, technical and assessment skills: • Gathering of data for clinical judgement, choice of examination, investigations and their interpretations. • Demonstrating proficiency in performing physical examinations and using diagnostic and therapeutic instruments.	Positive indicators: • Asks open questions (to explore work issues) followed by closed questions to clarify the extent of depressive symptoms. • Enquires about menopausal symptoms and explores their contribution to today's presentation. • Excludes red flags, such as ongoing postmenopausal bleeding and active suicidal ideation. Negative indicators: • Questioning is not selective. Most questions should be about 'bullying at work'; 'menopausal low mood' should be ruled out. • Doctors are too focused on the bio-medical aspects. • Doctors appear disorganised or fail to explain why they ask certain questions (menopause, PMB, suicide risk).
B. Clinical management skills • Recognition and management of common medical conditions in primary care. Demonstrates flexible and structured approach to decision-making. • Demonstrating ability to deal with multiple complaints and co-morbidity and to promote a shared approach to managing problems.	Positive indicators: • Doctors explain clearly what they feel is the appropriate diagnosis and verbalise their reasoning to the patient. • Management options, including occupational advice, are openly discussed and offered to the patient. • Management, including any prescription, is appropriate to the patient's level of risk. Negative indicators: • Doctors fail to make an adequate diagnosis, namely 'mild to moderate depression with a low suicide risk'. • Management plans, including prescribing, are not appropriate or in line with current best practice. • Follow-up arrangements are inadequate.

C. Interpersonal skills	Positive indicators:
• Use of recognised communication techniques that enhance understanding of a patient's illness and promote a shared approach to managing problems. • Practising ethically with respect for equality and diversity in line with accepted codes of professional conduct.	• Doctors display good listening skills; they identify the patient's dilemma and fears. • They develop a *shared* management plan, which incorporates the patient's specific concerns about work. • Time off work and follow-up is skilfully negotiated. Negative indicators: • Doctors interrupt inappropriately; appear judgemental or doctor-centred. • Formulaic questions are employed; the questioning on depressive symptoms sounds like a reading of a questionnaire. • Doctors fail to empathise with how this problem has changed the patient's life and her self-perception.

Group debrief

- Assess the doctor's verbal and non-verbal response to the patient requesting a sick note. Did the doctor seem genuinely interested and respectful? Was touch used overly and out of context?
- Was the consultation 'clunky' and lacking in natural flow? Were rote questions and phrases used? Was the patient given time to answer questions? Were questions replicated and old ground covered repeatedly? Did the doctor feel confident, once sufficient data were gathered for a diagnosis, to move smoothly on to management?
- Was there a shared management plan that incorporated the patient's concerns and expectations?
- The most common reason for failure in the CSA is that the doctor 'does not develop a management plan (including prescribing and referral) that is appropriate and in line with current best practice or make adequate arrangements for follow-up and safety-netting'. Evaluate whether the management of this case (mild–moderate depression) was correct, safe and broad enough to eliminate the differential (menopause)?

Relevant literature

For clinical guidance on depression, see www.cks.nhs.uk/depression

For advice on bullying from the Advisory, Conciliation and Arbitration Service (ACAS), see www.acas.org.uk/index.aspx?articleid=1864

Practice case 7 - Blood test results

Brief to the patient

- You are Evelyn Baker, a 35 year old housewife.
- You present today to discuss the results of a recent blood test. If questioned in detail, you had the 'lucozade test' because a fasting glucose test two months ago showed you had borderline diabetes. You also requested your cholesterol be checked because you are hoping to stop the cholesterol medication.
- You deliberately, without telling the doctor, did not take your cholesterol tablets for one month preceding the blood test in the hope that if the level is low, your doctor will stop the cholesterol tablet. You give this information to the doctor only when your blood results are being discussed.
- With your diet and exercise programme over the last year, you lost a stone and hope a healthy lifestyle will enable you to discontinue medication. You do not experience side effects from medication.
- You think that you may develop diabetes in future. Your mother's parents developed late onset diabetes in their forties. Your father had a heart attack in his fifties and your mother had one in her sixties. Three of your mother's uncles and her only sister have high cholesterol.
- You expect the doctor to discuss your results and to stop the tablets if your cholesterol is low. You also expect your medication for heavy periods to be re-issued today. The gynaecologist you saw two weeks ago advised an operation to burn out the lining of the womb but until then, you need medication to ease the bleeding.
- You are worried about being lectured about further weight loss. You think you have 'big bones' and a 'slow metabolism' and it took enormous effort to lose weight over the last year. You are tired of being warned about the risks of being overweight. You are a non-smoker. You and your husband share three bottles of white wine each week.
- If the doctor offers further blood tests or referral to a specialist, you want to know why.

Patient medical record for the doctor

Name   Evelyn Baker (35 years)

Past medical history   Iron deficiency anaemia 2008
                            Menorrhagia 2008
                            Latex allergy 2007

This practice case originally appeared in *GP* and is reproduced here in an amended form with permission (see www.gponline.com)

Current medication	Simvastatin 40 mg at night
	Mefenamic acid 500 mg three times daily
	Tranexamic acid 1 g three times daily

Blood tests	Tests done two weeks ago
Fasting glucose	6.5 mmol/l
Two-hour glucose	10.8 mmol/l
Serum cholesterol	5.9 mmol/l (three years ago 7.9 mmol/l)
HDL	1.1 mmol/l
Hb	13.9 g/dl
BP	136/86
BMI	34.7

Marking guide for the assessor

Generic indicators for targeted assessment domains	Descriptors – positive and negative
A. Data gathering, technical and assessment skills: • Gathering of data for clinical judgement, choice of examination, investigations and their interpretations. • Demonstrating proficiency in performing physical examinations and using diagnostic and therapeutic instruments.	Positive indicators: • Finds out what the patient already knows about the blood tests and why they were done. • Discusses the patient's ideas about cholesterol and explores her beliefs regarding treatment. • Discovers the patient's expectation of discontinuing with simvastatin and obtaining a repeat prescription for menorrhagia medication. • The patient is examined for clinical signs of hypercholesterolaemia Negative indicators: • Does not explore her family history. • Time is wasted on examinations that contribute little to subsequent management plans.

B. Clinical management skills	Positive indicators:
• Recognition and management of common medical conditions in primary care. Demonstrates flexible and structured approach to decision-making. • Demonstrating ability to deal with multiple complaints and comorbidity and to promote a shared approach to managing problems.	• Negotiates and highlights the four main issues: her new diagnosis of impaired glucose tolerance, the possibility of familial hypercholesterolaemia, the risks and benefits of statin therapy, and a brief review of menorrhagia management prior to prescribing. • Addresses her concerns about unnecessary statin intake and manages in line with national policy. • The repeat prescription is issued with clear instructions, in line with national prescribing guidance. • Adequate follow-up is arranged and the doctor checks that the patient understands why future tests or referrals are needed. Negative indicators: • Fails to interpret the results appropriately, or the decision regarding statin therapy is not justified. • Prescribes inappropriately. • Follow-up arrangements are inadequate.
C. Interpersonal skills	Positive indicators:
• Use of recognised communication techniques that enhance understanding of a patient's illness and promote a shared approach to managing problems. • Practising ethically with respect for equality and diversity in line with accepted codes of professional conduct.	• Understands why she discontinued medication prior to the blood test. • Provides information about CV risk in language that is easily understood. Explanations are concise. • Provides opportunities for the patient to seek clarification. • Offers options and involves the patient in management decisions. Negative indicators: • Adopts a 'parent–child' style of consulting. • Delivers standard health promotion advice without tailoring it to this patient's needs.

Group debrief

- The focus of some CSA cases is data interpretation. In this case, the patient's blood results are provided for interpretation. You need to interpret the results correctly. Sometimes candidates interpret the results correctly but then fail to act on them appropriately. Examiners therefore conclude that the candidate did not recognise their significance. It is imperative to deal with abnormal findings safely, in line with national or local guidance to reduce risk.
- When candidates fail to interpret data correctly, they invariably do not make the correct working diagnosis. Making a diagnosis means committing yourself on the basis of the information you have available to you. You need a sound knowledge-base.
- State the diagnosis clearly and explain it to the patient using language that is understandable. The lack of a statement about the diagnosis and a vague summary leaves the examiner wondering whether you have made a diagnosis at all. In this case, evaluate how well the doctor explained impaired glucose tolerance and the possibility of familial hypercholesterolaemia to the patient.
- To assess the doctor's interpersonal skills, consider whether the doctor worked in partnership with the patient, involved her in management decisions, and demonstrated evidence of 'shared understanding' by asking the patient to summarise what she understood?

Relevant literature

Choudhary F., Al-Hadithy H. & Simon C. (2009) Hypercholesterolaemia. *InnovAiT*, **2(12):** 721–31.

DeMott K., Nherera L., Shaw E.J. *et al.* (2008) *Familial hypercholesterolaemia: the identification and management of adults and children with familial hypercholesterolaemia.* London: National Collaborating Centre for Primary Care and Royal College of General Practitioners. www.nice.org.uk/nicemedia/live/12048/41700/41700.pdf

Wylie G. *et al.* (2002) Impaired glucose tolerance: qualitative and quantitative study of general practitioners' knowledge and perceptions. *BMJ*, **324:** 1190.

Clinical Knowledge Summaries (www.cks.nhs.uk/home) are a useful resource.

Practice case 8 – A list of problems

Brief to the patient

- You are Lorraine Brooker, a 28 year old accountant, married and in your tenth week of pregnancy.
- You have come to see the doctor today because you have been troubled by headaches, a cold that won't go away, morning sickness, sluggish bowels and thinning hair. You have written a list of your symptoms. Your opening statement is 'I'm so forgetful these days. I brought a list of problems with me.'
- If asked which symptom is most troublesome, you say all the symptoms are troublesome but the headaches are the worst because they have been present for two weeks, since the onset of your cold. The boring pain behind your right eye affects work. The teeth on the right side of your mouth ache. When questioned in detail, you admit to having hot and cold spells at night, an offensive post-nasal drip and your forehead pain worsens when you bend forward.
- You want to know if it is worth buying £12 acupressure bracelets for the nausea you have throughout the day.
- Your bowel pattern has altered from once daily to once every two to three days.
- You have always had fine hair but when your cousin was recently diagnosed with a thyroid problem, you checked the internet for advice.
- You think you have a recurrence of migraine (you had this as a teenager). You are concerned about coping with tax season at work with these headaches.
- You want to discuss all your problems. Medication for the headache and a blood test for thyroid disease is a priority. If asked, you are not allergic to any antibiotics.
- If examined, you do not have a temperature and you are tender over the right eye.

Patient medical record for the doctor

Name   Lorraine Brooker (28 years)

Past medical history   Currently pregnant
                            Irritable bowel syndrome

Past medication   Mebeverine

This practice case originally appeared in *GP* and is reproduced here in an amended form with permission (see www.gponline.com)

Marking guide for the assessor

Generic indicators for targeted assessment domains	Descriptors – positive and negative
A. Data gathering, technical and assessment skills: • Gathering of data for clinical judgement, choice of examination, investigations and their interpretations. • Demonstrating proficiency in performing physical examinations and using diagnostic and therapeutic instruments.	Positive indicators: • Asks open questions (to explore the list's contents) followed by closed questions to clarify details, particularly of the headache. • Enquires about the past history of migraine. Understands how pressures at work (and her cousin's recent diagnosis with thyroid disease) affect her presentation today. • The targeted examination is focused, practised and integrated into the consultation. Negative indicators: • Fails to identify the patient's agenda and preferences. • Makes assumptions (about migraine/minor pregnancy symptoms) and fails to recognise the challenge. • Is disorganised in gathering information.
B. Clinical management skills • Recognition and management of common medical conditions in primary care. Demonstrates flexible and structured approach to decision-making. • Demonstrating ability to deal with multiple complaints and co-morbidity and to promote a shared approach to managing problems.	Positive indicators: • Candidates explain clearly what they want to examine and why. • The risks and benefits of management options, including prescribing, are adequately discussed. • Candidates' responses to the patient's concerns and expectations are smoothly woven into the consultation. Negative indicators: • By failing to make an adequate diagnosis, the candidates' explanation to the patient is vague or lacks clarity. • Management plans, including prescribing, are not appropriate or in line with current best practice. • Follow-up arrangements are inadequate.

C. Interpersonal skills	Positive indicators:
• Use of recognised communication techniques that enhance understanding of a patient's illness and promote a shared approach to managing problems. • Practising ethically with respect for equality and diversity in line with accepted codes of professional conduct.	• Displays good listening skills; appears genuinely interested in getting to the heart of the problem. • Develops a *shared* management plan, incorporating the patient's agenda and specific concerns. • Checks understanding and agreement with the patient. Negative indicators: • Interrupts inappropriately, appears judgemental or lacks sympathy • Uses formulaic questions; the consultation lacks natural flow. • Is doctor-centred; fails to adequately pick up or address verbal or non-verbal cues.

Group debrief

- Assess the doctor's verbal and non-verbal response to the patient presenting with a list. In the opening moments of the consultation, did the doctor seem genuinely interested in ascertaining the main reason for the patient consulting today?
- Was there a good mix of open and closed questions to adequately and safely prioritise the focus of the consultation?
- Was the consultation over-modelled using rote questions? Were the questions used to elicit the patient's agenda appropriately interwoven into the consultation?
- Was there a shared management plan? Did the doctor elicit and address Lorraine's idea that she had a migraine, her concern that she will be unable to cope with work because of the headache, and her expectation of a blood test for thyroid disease?
- One of the most common feedback statements to CSA failures is 'does not identify the patient's agenda, health beliefs and preferences or does not make use of verbal and non-verbal cues.' In this case, evaluate whether the doctor remained attentive and curious to a patient presenting with a list. The skill in this case is to show competent use of listening skills while remaining aware of the consultation's challenges from the doctor's perspective.

Relevant literature

Suchman A.L. *et al.* (1997) A model of empathic communication in the medical interview. *JAMA*, **277(8):** 678–682.

Search www.skillscascade.com/index.html for articles on agenda setting and patient cues.

Practice case 9 – Pruritis in pregnancy

Brief to the patient

- You are Becky Engels, a 28 year old married woman. You are currently 32 weeks pregnant with your first baby. It has been an uneventful pregnancy so far.
- You have come to see the doctor today because you have had a severe 'all over' itch for the last three days. E45 didn't help. If questioned in detail, the itch is worse over your hands and feet, but there is nothing to see.
- You have not been in contact with anything new and you have not come into contact with chickenpox. You don't feel unwell.
- You think the itchiness may be a reaction to the powdered gloves you use at work. You work for a dental laboratory making dentures. Work switched from powdered to non-powdered gloves 4 years ago but you think you are having a delayed reaction to latex.
- You are also having a stressful time at work. Your pregnant work colleague is being allowed to start her maternity leave at 32 weeks because she has symphysis pubis pain. You have been asked to start leave at 38 weeks.
- If offered, you are concerned about using steroid creams and Piriton while pregnant. You would like a week off work because you are tired and the itch is disrupting your sleep.
- If the doctor offers a blood test or hospital referral, you want to know why. You become concerned that something is wrong. What should you tell your husband? Will you have to start maternity leave soon? What should you tell work?

Patient medical record for the doctor

Name   Rebecca Engels (28 years)

Past medical history   Currently pregnant

Current medication   none

This practice case originally appeared in *GP* and is reproduced here in an amended form with permission (see www.gponline.com)

Marking guide for the assessor

Generic indicators for targeted assessment domains	Descriptors – positive and negative
A. Data gathering, technical and assessment skills: • Gathering of data for clinical judgement, choice of examination, investigations and their interpretations. • Demonstrating proficiency in performing physical examinations and using diagnostic and therapeutic instruments.	Positive indicators: • Gets details of itch – asks about jaundice, pale stools, possible viral hepatitis. Checks that mum is feeling well and baby is kicking. • Finds out the patient's ideas about possible latex allergy or sensitivity to powdered gloves and explains why this is unlikely. • Elicits relevant work stressors. • Discovers the patient's expectations for topical treatment and time off work. Negative indicators: • Fails to elicit above points. • Assumes this is dry skin or eczema.
B. Clinical management skills • Recognition and management of common medical conditions in primary care. Demonstrates flexible and structured approach to decision-making. • Demonstrating ability to deal with multiple complaints and co-morbidity and to promote a shared approach to managing problems.	Positive indicators: • Explains the possibility of bile-salt pruritis in pregnancy using jargon-free language, without alarming the patient. • Addresses her concerns about Piriton and steroid creams. If prescribes, the medication is appropriate and evidence based, with clear instructions on how to use and its safety in pregnancy. • Makes balanced plans: requests the appropriate blood tests (bile salts, LFTs, viral screen), liaises with the midwife or refers directly to obstetrics, in line with local policy. Negative indicators: • Fails to elicit above points. • Fails to explain the management plan clearly or alarms the patient inappropriately. • Prescribes inappropriately.

C. Interpersonal skills	Positive indicators:
• Use of recognised communication techniques that enhance understanding of a patient's illness and promote a shared approach to managing problems. • Practising ethically with respect for equality and diversity in line with accepted codes of professional conduct.	• Displays empathy to her work situation • Advises her on what she should tell her husband and her work. • Involves the patient in decisions about blood tests, midwife, or hospital referral. Negative indicators: • Fails to elicit above points • Is underly or overly challenging when negotiating time off work. • Makes judgemental or non-professional statements about her boss, colleagues, or midwife.

Group debrief

- Evaluate whether the doctor gathered sufficient information, from the history and examination, to arrive at a reasonable hypothesis regarding the cause of this patient's itchiness. Were red flags, such as anorexia, jaundice, a bruising tendency and a reduction in foetal movements excluded?
- Did the doctor elicit and address Becky's idea about latex allergy causing her itch; her concerns about the medication or illness harming the baby; and her expectation of a sick note?
- Did the doctor explain the diagnosis and management plan in jargon-free language? Did he refer for specialist advice, discuss that certain blood tests were needed and that closer monitoring of the baby may be needed? Did he provide the information in chunks and check the patient's understanding at each step?
- Evaluate whether the doctor handled the request for a sick note fairly and dealt with the maternity leave issue in a way that encouraged the patient's autonomy.
- Did the doctor involve the patient in decisions and offer the patient options? In some cases, it may be difficult to offer choice, as in this case where a referral to obstetrics is warranted. The doctor could say, 'I think that the safest thing to do is organise blood tests and monitoring of the baby in hospital. How do you feel about that?' This allows the patient to voice any reasons why she cannot go to hospital (such as 'there is nobody at home to look after my step-son when he returns from school'. However, involving the patient in the decision-making provides the opportunity to uncover and deal with potential problems.

Relevant literature

www.gpnotebook.co.uk – search for 'raised bile acids in pregnancy'.

Practice case 10 – UTI in a young man

Brief to the patient

- You are Jake Gibson, a 29 year old married man.
- You have come to see the doctor today because for the last 24 hours, you have been going to the toilet every 1 to 2 hours. You have a 'burning feeling' when you pass urine.
- If questioned in detail, you deny feeling unwell or having a high fever. You do not have diarrhoea or vomiting but you have mild nausea that has prevented you from eating today. You haven't had kidney stones, loin pain or frothy or bloodstained urine.
- If asked, you have not been unfaithful to your wife. Both of you had negative 'VD' screens before commencing your relationship.
- You think you have a bladder infection. When your wife had similar symptoms, she was given a short course of antibiotics.
- You have just been to the toilet while in the waiting room and you definitely cannot produce a urine sample now. You also have an urgent appointment with your bank manager and will find it difficult to return to the surgery later.
- You are a snowboarding instructor for an events company and leave in three days for a 2-week snowboarding job in Austria. You don't know what medical facilities are available at the resort.
- You want some antibiotics, just like your wife was given. You are not allergic to any antibiotics.
- If you are told to bring a sample back, you become impatient because you were told the blood tests and kidney scans done in April last year ruled out any kidney problems.

Patient medical record for the doctor

Name   Jake Gibson (29 years)

Past medical history   Isolated microscopic haematuria (April last year)

Letter from nephrologist (April last year):

'Dear GP
I do not feel that low level microscopic haematuria in the absence of proteinuria, abnormal renal function, hypertension or symptoms requires further investigation.

This practice case originally appeared in *GP* and is reproduced here in an amended form with permission (see **www.gponline.com**)

243

You may consider arranging an ultrasound. I am sure this is likely to be normal but it is conceivable that you may pick up dysplastic, atrophic or polycystic kidneys. I do not think a renal appointment will add anything.'

Investigations

U&Es (April):	No abnormality
US kidneys (April):	Normal appearances. Both kidneys normal size. No pc dilatation. Normal bladder.

Marking guide for the assessor

Generic indicators for targeted assessment domains	Descriptors – positive and negative
A. Data gathering, technical and assessment skills: • Gathering of data for clinical judgement, choice of examination, investigations and their interpretations. • Demonstrating proficiency in performing physical examinations and using diagnostic and therapeutic instruments.	Positive indicators: • Systematically works through a diagnostic sieve: UTI, STI and kidney stones. • Enquires about Jake's previous investigation for recurrent microscopic haematuria. Understands how Jake's previous negative investigation and his wife's UTI treatment affect his presentation today. • Asks for a urine sample. Note – in the absence of symptoms of systemic illness, marks are not deducted if a more detailed physical examination is omitted. Negative indicators: • Fails to elicit above points. • Assumes this is a UTI; does not take a sexual history.

B. Clinical management skills	Positive indicators:
• Recognition and management of common medical conditions in primary care. Demonstrates flexible and structured approach to decision-making. • Demonstrating ability to deal with multiple complaints and co-morbidity and to promote a shared approach to managing problems.	• Persuades the patient to drop off an MSU and discusses potential management plans based on either positive or negative results. • If prescribes, chooses a suitable antibiotic (at correct dose and duration) with clear instructions on how to take the medication. If he tries to negotiate a delayed prescription or no prescription, justifies his reasoning. • Provides information about UTIs in men and how their investigation and management differs from UTIs in women. Negative indicators: • Fails to elicit above points. • By failing to adequately explain why an MSU is important, the patient remains unaware or unconvinced of the dangers of not returning with an MSU.
C. Interpersonal skills	Positive indicators:
• Use of recognised communication techniques that enhance understanding of a patient's illness and promote a shared approach to managing problems. • Practising ethically with respect for equality and diversity in line with accepted codes of professional conduct.	• Shows flexibility and empathy – arranges investigations and treatment around the patient's work commitments. • Involves the patient in decisions, negotiates an MSU and follow-up. • In explaining UTIs in men, uses the patient's ideas about 'bladder infections' and builds on what the patient already knows about the treatment of UTIs in women. Negative indicators: • Fails to elicit above points. • Is didactic – hastily recommends Jake cancel or postpone his trip. • Is rigid – lacks sensitivity to the patient's tight timescales.

Group debrief

- Did the doctor elicit and address Jake's idea that there is no difference in the treatment of UTIs in men and women; his concern that further (repetitive) investigations will unnecessarily delay his work trip; and his expectation of immediate antibiotics?
- Did the doctor adequately explain the need for an MSU?
- Evaluate the doctor's response to Jake's reluctance to return later with an MSU. Was he sensitive to Jake's pressured deadlines?
- Evaluate whether the doctor dealt adequately with the uncertainty created by not having an MSU. Was he safe in his management?
- The most common feedback statement to CSA failures is 'does not develop a management plan (including prescription and referral) that is appropriate and in line with current best practice or make arrangements for follow-up and safety netting'. In this case, evaluate whether the doctor formulated a safe management plan for a patient who perceives further investigation as repetitive and time-consuming. The skill in this case is to shift the patient's ideas so that he wants to be investigated further and prioritises getting an MSU to the surgery before leaving on his overseas trip.

Relevant literature

www.sign.ac.uk/pdf/sign88.pdf – pages 16–17.

Practice case 11 – Sexual problems

Brief to the patient

- You are Robert Williams, a 64 year old engineer, looking forward to your retirement and move to Spain in 3 months.
- You present today, slightly embarrassed but determined, to ask for a prescription of Viagra.
- Your wife died two years ago. You started dating a 54-year-old divorcee, Fiona, three months ago. You have a good relationship but when you attempted a sexual relationship last weekend, you were unable to maintain your erection. This happened twice for the first time last weekend.
- If asked, you say that you still get erections at night. You have never suffered from premature ejaculation. Your libido during your last year of marriage was reduced because, you suspect, your wife was very unwell with bowel cancer.
- You and Fiona have talked. You find her attractive. You are not suffering from grief or guilt. Your mood is fine. Your grown-up children like Fiona. You are financially secure.
- You think that you have 'performance anxiety' and if you take 'Viagra', which you read about on the internet, you will feel confident, you will sustain a good erection and once the cycle is broken, you will not require further medication.
- If asked, you are in good health, currently asymptomatic and you have not had previous medical issues or surgery. You are not taking any medication, except for the occasional ibuprofen for back pain. You have no problems with urine flow or frequency. You do not know your family history, having been adopted.
- In the last two years, you have eaten more ready meals, put on 10kg, drink 4 beers three times per week and a bottle of red wine on weekends. You smoke the occasional cigar. You do very little exercise.
- If the doctor asks to examine your BP and weight, you hand him a card: 'BP 134/86'; 'weight 90kg; BMI 29'. If an examination of the genitalia is requested, hand over a card: 'normal penis and testes'. If the doctor asks to examine your prostate, decline, deferring this.
- You want a prescription of Viagra, preferably an NHS script, but you are resigned to paying for it. You are worried about the quality of the tablets sold on the internet. You want the script today because you have planned a romantic weekend away.

This practice case originally appeared in *GP* and is reproduced here in an amended form with permission (see **www.gponline.com**)

Patient medical record for the doctor

Name   Robert Williams (64 years)

Past medical history   Mechanical low back pain (2009) – sick note × 1 week

Fungal nail infection (2005)

Marking guide for the assessor

Generic indicators for targeted assessment domains	Descriptors – positive and negative
A. Data gathering, technical and assessment skills: • Gathering of data for clinical judgement, choice of examination, investigations and their interpretations. • Demonstrating proficiency in performing physical examinations and using diagnostic and therapeutic instruments.	Positive indicators: • Asks open questions (to explore the medication request and type of sexual problem) followed by closed questions to clarify possible causes of erectile dysfunction (ED) such as CV, depression, endocrine, surgical, medication side effect or psychological issues such as family or financial anxieties. • Enquires about lifestyle: smoking, alcohol, exercise and diet. • Undertakes a targeted examination: BP, weight, penis and testes. In the absence of lower urinary tract symptoms, a prostate examination is deferred. Negative indicators: • Questioning is not sufficiently detailed to exclude organic or psychological causes of ED. • In particular, the opportunity to explore cardiovascular issues and question holistically (job, children, grief) is missed. • The physical examination is not undertaken or is insufficiently targeted.

B. Clinical management skills	Positive indicators:
• Recognition and management of common medical conditions in primary care. Demonstrates flexible and structured approach to decision-making. • Demonstrating ability to deal with multiple complaints and co-morbidity and to promote a shared approach to managing problems.	• Doctors discuss further investigation and justify their request for blood tests (fasting glucose, lipids, thyroid, UandEs, FBC, thyroid and possibly serum testosterone). • Management options, including delaying prescription until completion of investigation or writing a private prescription, are openly discussed and offered to the patient. • If new medication is prescribed, the patient is advised on safe dosing and cautioned about possible side effects. • Adequate follow-up is arranged. Negative indicators: • The investigation of the problem is inadequate or poorly targeted. • Doctors prescribe medication for ED on the NHS, out of line with current guidance. • If prescribed medication on a private script, patients are inadequately advised about dose, timing, need for sexual stimulation or likelihood of success. • Follow-up arrangements are inadequate.

C. Interpersonal skills	Positive indicators:
• Use of recognised communication techniques that enhance understanding of a patient's illness and promote a shared approach to managing problems. • Practising ethically with respect for equality and diversity in line with accepted codes of professional conduct.	• Doctors deal sensitively with a potentially embarrassing problem. Questions are asked in a professional manner. • The examination and management is conducted with confidence. • Information about further investigation is delivered concisely, in language that is easily understood. • The patient is provided with opportunities to seek clarification. Negative indicators: • The doctor assumes the patient wants an NHS script and becomes inappropriately confrontational. • The doctor does not encourage the patient to share his ideas and is inappropriately doctor-centred. • The doctor does not negotiate a mutually acceptable plan.

Group debrief

- Some CSA cases are written with the patient asking for something specific. In this case, the patient asks for Viagra. In other cases, the patient may ask for a referral or a blood test or a procedure, such as a vasectomy. The importance in such cases to explore the patient's reasons for the request.
- It is also imperative to assess if alternative options, which the patient may not have considered, are more appropriate. In this case, marks are awarded if attention is paid to modifying the patient's lifestyle and assessing his CV risk as well as negotiating the Viagra prescription.
- A common reason for failure in the CSA is the doctor 'does not recognise the challenge (e.g. the patient's problem or ethical dilemma)'. Evaluate whether the doctor adequately explored the patient's problem by asking sufficient questions about organic and psycho-social issues. Did the patient ascertain the patient's ideas and redress his expectations by discussing the limited success rate of the requested medication? Evaluate whether the ethical dilemma (who pays for the medication) was negotiated in a supportive and sensitive manner.

Relevant literature

British Society for Sexual Medicine (2007) *Guidelines on the Management of Erectile Dysfunction*: www.bssm.org.uk

McMahon C.N., Smith C.J. & Shabsigh R. (2006) Treating erectile dysfunction when PDE5 inhibitors fail, *BMJ*, **332:** 589–592.

Practice case 12 – Scanty periods

Brief to the patient

- You are Polly Avery, a 28 year old administrative assistant at a local timber merchants, unmarried and single for the last three years.
- You attend today because when you saw the practice nurse for a smear last week, she advised you that it is not good for your health to have only three periods in a year, but she was unable to explain why this is a problem.
- If questioned about how the problem started, you are not sure. You stopped taking the combined pill (Cileste) three years ago. For the first two years, your periods occurred every two months. In the last year, you had a period every four months. Bleeding is light and unpredictable. You are not troubled by the irregular bleeding and until the nurse mentioned it, had not perceived a problem.
- If specifically questioned, you admit to hair growing on your chest and chin, which you remove. You have an oily T-zone but no acne.
- Despite playing rugby, running to keep fit, and attendance at a weekly slimming club, you find it difficult to lose the 12kg you gained three years ago after your relationship ended.
- If asked, you do not have symptoms of diabetes – no excessive thirst or urination or recurrent minor infections.
- You are not in a relationship and fertility is currently not an issue.
- You had ignored these symptoms of scanty, infrequent periods, difficulty losing weight and excessive hairiness on your chin and chest, but the nurse's reaction scared you into asking yourself whether you have a gynaecological problem. Are tests needed? What can you do to improve your health?
- If a family history is taken, you say that your family is healthy, but if polycystic ovarian syndrome (PCOS) is mentioned, you recall that your sister (age 40) may have this. You know very little about PCOS, but you are keen to know more. You would like to read some written information before deciding on a particular treatment.
- If tests are ordered, you want to know what the results could mean. You are concerned that these will affect your insurance. You plan to buy a house soon.
- If weight loss is mentioned, you sigh and appear defeated. It has been a struggle to keep the weight off over the last three years and you are not hopeful about losing more weight.
- If the doctor examines you, the card you hand to him or her states 'BP 134/88, pulse 86, weight 87 kg; BMI 28'.

Patient medical record for the doctor

Name   Polly Avery (28 years)

Past medical history   Thoracic back pain 3 months ago
                               Ankle pain from rugby injury 9 months ago

Past medication   Diclofenac 50 mg thrice daily (9 months ago)
                               Omeprazole 20 mg once daily (9 months ago)

Consultation note by Practice Nurse (last week):
'LMP 12 of last month. No previous smear abnormalities. Very irregular menstrual cycle. 4–5 months between periods. Not currently sexually active. Never smoked tobacco.
O/E: medium speculum. Transition zone seen. Smear taken. Nullip – bled slightly on contact. BP 132/80.
Plan: will write to patient with smear results. Advised to see GP to discuss periods.'

Marking guide for the assessor

Generic indicators for targeted assessment domains	Descriptors – positive and negative
A. Data gathering, technical and assessment skills: • Gathering of data for clinical judgement, choice of examination, investigations and their interpretations. • Demonstrating proficiency in performing physical examinations and using diagnostic and therapeutic instruments.	Positive indicators: • Makes use of the medical record provided and gathers sufficient information through the use of open and closed questions to suspect PCOS. • Excludes red flags – asks about other metabolic problems such as diabetes. • The doctor is holistic – marital status, plans for a family, and occupation are discussed. • The doctor performs a general examination relevant to supporting or refuting the diagnosis of PCOS. Negative indicators: • Does not systematically gather data from history or examination; makes assumptions about the problem. • Not appropriately selective in choice of examination. • Fails to interpret examination findings correctly.

B. Clinical management skills	Positive indicators:
• Recognition and management of common medical conditions in primary care. Demonstrates flexible and structured approach to decision-making. • Demonstrating ability to deal with multiple complaints and co-morbidity and to promote a shared approach to managing problems.	• The doctor on the basis of probability makes a diagnosis of PCOS. • The explanation of PCOS is in simple, jargon-free language. The doctor checks the patient's understanding periodically. • Management options, including possible blood tests, scans or referral to the practice nurse for nutritional support, are openly discussed. • Management is evidence based and informed by UK guidelines. Negative indicators: • The doctor fails to consider common causes of oligomenorrhoea. • The doctor fails to sufficiently explain what PCOS is to enhance the patient's understanding. • Further investigation and management is not appropriate or inappropriately timed (urgent rather than routine tests are requested). • Follow-up arrangements are inadequate.

C. Interpersonal skills	Positive indicators:
• Use of recognised communication techniques that enhance understanding of a patient's illness and promote a shared approach to managing problems. • Practising ethically with respect for equality and diversity in line with accepted codes of professional conduct.	• Enquires about why the patient presents today – her concerns and expectations are elicited at an early stage. • The doctor shares his or her thoughts and involves the patient in decisions. • By providing explanations that are relevant and understandable, the patient's autonomy and opinions are encouraged. Hence, the management plan, including the possible prescription of hormonal medication, is jointly constructed. • The cue about difficulties with weight is recognised and the doctor responds appropriately. Negative indicators: • The doctor makes assumptions from reading the nurse's notes and fails to inquire about the patient's health understanding or respond to her concerns. • The doctor fails to explore the patient's psychosocial context and assumes that fertility or fears about diabetes drive her presentation today. • The doctor fails to inform or empower the patient to contribute to management decisions; a prescription for hormonal medication or a list for a battery of tests is handed to the patient with inadequate explanation. • The doctor fails to recognise or respond to the cue about weight.

Group debrief

- The most common reason for failure in the CSA is the candidate's failure to develop a management plan.
- This case tests the candidate's ability to recognise and manage the first presentation of oligomenorrhoea. The history taking and examination should be sufficiently selective to arrive at a possible diagnosis of PCOS fairly quickly. It is important to establish which aspect of PCOS will be the priority for treatment. Fertility, hirsutism, diabetes and hypertension are not identified as pressing problems. However, the doctor is aware of the relationship between oligomenorrhoea and endometrial cancer – this aspect of care is prioritised so subsequent discussion about treatment addresses the need to induce withdrawal bleeds every 3–4 months.
- Assess how well the candidate discussed 'PCOS and having very infrequent periods'. Was the explanation jargon-free or did it sound technical or alarming to the patient? Did the doctor discuss possible blood tests or scans? Did the patient understand why these investigations were being requested?
- Did the doctor involve the patient in decisions and offer the patient options? This patient had an expectation of being given information about the condition before deciding on a treatment pathway. Was the doctor able to elicit and respond to this expectation? Or, did the doctor ignore this expectation and try to prescribe in this first consultation a treatment to induce withdrawal bleeds?
- What was the doctor's response to the weight cue? How empathetic was the response? Was the doctor's response 'patient education' or the giving of information, somewhat authoritarian? Or did the doctor try to explore the patient's motivation to lose weight? When the patient revealed her difficulties, was the doctor's response neutral, for example: 'How do you make sense of all of this?' and appropriately reflective: 'Do you see a way to increase your exercise or reduce your calories?'? The high-scoring candidate in the 'Interpersonal Skills' section demonstrates good motivational interviewing skills: an open style that allows the patient to explore her strategies for overcoming barriers to change; agenda setting; open questions; reflective listening and affirmations.

Relevant literature

For an excellent overview of the management of PCOS, see:
Harding E (2010) Polycystic Ovarian Syndrome, *InnovAiT*, **3 (2):** 71–75.
doi: 10.1093/innovait/inp124

To develop your motivational interviewing skills, see:
Storr E (2011) Motivational interviewing: a positive approach, *InnovAiT,* **4(9):** 533–538.
doi:10.1093/innovait/inr045

Practice case 13 – Harmful alcohol intake

Brief to the patient

- You are Martin Stander, a 28 year old unmarried man who works as a coordinator for a local logistics company. You attend to ask the doctor for a referral to the practice counsellor for 'help with my drinking'.

- Your drinking has increased over the last six weeks and you have got into trouble twice with the police. On these two occasions, you got into fights and on the last occasion you had to be restrained, hence the bruises on your face today. The police hearings are set for a week and a month away. The police have told you that you are 'throwing your life and career away'. You want to take their advice and seek help with your drinking.

- The fights were unprovoked. Nobody was seriously injured because you 'lose all coordination when drunk'.

- If specifically asked whom you are angry with, you say 'with life and circumstances'. Your girlfriend is 4 months pregnant with your child. You feel uncertain about getting married and think you are too young to become a father. You feel angry about the contraception failure.

- Your girlfriend plans to move in with you into your parents' house because you cannot afford to live on your own. Your parents have been supportive. Although you haven't decided to marry as yet, you feel your mum will become attached to the baby and it will be difficult to part ways after the baby's birth. Your girlfriend, after the last fight, asked if you wanted her to move out. You are working things through. You have been in a steady relationship for 11 months. Your girlfriend attends the local teacher training college. Her family live two hours' drive away.

- Your older brother married young (age 19) and divorced three years later. He has experienced difficulty in seeing his children. Your mother often says she feels sad that her grandchildren 'are strangers to her'.

- You are a good rugby player and your social life revolves around the local rugby club. You usually binge after rugby matches, but restrict your intake to less than 20 units per week. Over the last 6 weeks, you drank 'way more than this' and try to pass out so you don't have to think about your situation.

- Your main symptom is anxiety about your future. You do not have symptoms of depression – no sleep disturbance, loss of appetite or weight, feelings of guilt or poor self-esteem or apathy or excessive tiredness.

- You would like to speak to someone 'to sort out my head' and you expect a referral to the practice counsellor.

- If the doctor discusses Alcoholics Anonymous with you, you say that you are not an alcoholic and don't think their service is appropriate to your needs.
- If signposted to local services (Relate or social services), you want to know how these services could be useful to you.
- If the doctor arranges a follow-up appointment, you want to know when and why you should attend. With the court appearances, you do not want to take too much time off work.

Patient medical record for the doctor

Name   Martin Stander (28 years)

Social and family history   Unmarried
                                Works for a logistics company
                                Plays 1st row for the local amateur rugby club

Past medical history   Hayfever (every spring)
                                Left AC joint injury (5 months ago)
                                Right ACL reconstruction (2 years ago)

Past medication   Loratidine 10mg daily (spring)

Marking guide for the assessor

Generic indicators for targeted assessment domains	Descriptors – positive and negative
A. Data gathering, technical and assessment skills: • Gathering of data for clinical judgement, choice of examination, investigations and their interpretations. • Demonstrating proficiency in performing physical examinations and using diagnostic and therapeutic instruments.	Positive indicators: • Asks selective questions, tailored to establishing whether hazardous drinking has occurred (e.g. FAST screening). Takes a comprehensive alcohol and drug history. • Checks if there are reasons (legal, occupational, insurance) why the patient may under-report alcohol consumption. Sufficient information is gathered to decide if adjunctive biological tests are needed. • Enquires about red flags, such as deliberate self-harm (DSH) and risk to others (domestic violence) from the patient's drinking. • Picks up the physical cue (facial bruise) – gathers information about recent fights / police involvement that leads to a deeper understanding of the patient's presentation today. • Details of the patient's support network are obtained. Negative indicators: • Questioning is not sufficiently selective. By the end of the history taking, the doctor is unable to quantify the extent of the drinking problem. • By the end of the history taking, the doctor is unable to decide whether adjunctive biological tests (GGT, MCV) are needed. • Assessment is not holistic – important information about work, hobbies (rugby) or family life (pregnant girlfriend moving in with mother who yearns for close relationship with grandchild) is missed.

B. Clinical management skills • Recognition and management of common medical conditions in primary care. Demonstrates flexible and structured approach to decision-making. • Demonstrating ability to deal with multiple complaints and co-morbidity and to promote a shared approach to managing problems.	Positive indicators: • The doctor makes a diagnosis – harmful drinking and using the patient's ideas and beliefs, feeds this back to the patient. • Management options, including abstinence or cutting down with goals of reduction, are jointly agreed. • While support networks and external agencies are discussed, the patient's personal responsibility for change is emphasised. • Review is planned: to offer encouragement, monitoring (MVC/GGT) or reassess (the costs and benefits of change). Negative indicators: • Doctors fail to manage safely or in line with current best practice. • Follow-up arrangements are inadequate.
C. Interpersonal skills • Use of recognised communication techniques that enhance understanding of a patient's illness and promote a shared approach to managing problems. • Practising ethically with respect for equality and diversity in line with accepted codes of professional conduct.	Positive indicators: • The doctor displays the skill of empathic interviewing: listening reflectively without cajoling or confronting; exploring with the patient the reasons for change as he sees his situation. • The doctor makes reflective statements and summarises periodically to check and convey understanding. • Personal responsibility is emphasised but the doctor supports the patient. • Statements are neutral and non-judgemental, thereby enhancing the patient's belief in their ability to change. Negative indicators: • The doctor does not listen attentively – seems distracted, pre-occupied or focused on uncovering a different (hidden) agenda. • The doctor gives advice, lectures or educates, potentially creating a parent–child dynamic. • The doctor appears judgemental or unhopeful about the patient's ability to change.

Group debrief

In this case, the doctor's main task is to empower the patient to self-care. On the surface, this appears to be a simple case – harmful alcohol usage. The patient's request for a referral to the practice counsellor is not unreasonable. The challenge in this case is the interpersonal skill – how good is the doctor at demonstrating skills to transform holistic understanding of the presenting problem into practical measures to move the patient forward? The motivational interviewing skills touched on in the previous case (PCOS) are also tested here.

With regard to interpersonal skills, assess whether the doctor:
- Asked questions to uncover relevant information outside the patient's current awareness: 'What might be the pros and cons of abstinence?'
- Accurate listening and empathic reflections: 'You sound confused about your girlfriend moving in with your parents.'
- Summarising/recapping information: 'to summarise what we have talked about so far...'
- Synthesising questions that ask the patient to apply the new information discovered to their original belief/behaviour: 'So on the one hand we talked about abstinence and on the other hand we spoke about cutting down. What do you make of it so far?'

Assess if the doctor, by the style of his or her consulting, strengthened the patient's desire to reduce drinking? Did the doctor make statements such as:
- What would you advise someone in your position to do?
- What would you do differently the next time you feel frustrated?
- How might we ensure this happens?
- How shall we handle any setbacks?

Relevant literature

Scottish Intercollegiate Guidelines Network (SIGN) (2003) The management of harmful drinking and alcohol dependence in primary care: www.sign.ac.uk/guidelines/fulltext/74/index.html.

For a brief overview on the philosophy of Motivational Interviewing and the stages of change, see: www.youtube.com/watch?v=4uUAELqp_9s. You can skip the first two minutes!

For an example of a five minute interview, see: www.youtube.com/watch?v=dm-rJJPCuTE.

Practice case 14 – Patient is peri-menopausal

Brief to the patient

- You are Kelly Carroll, a 46 year old woman. You present today, two weeks after having had some blood tests, to discuss the results. You definitely fasted for the blood test.
- The doctor who requested the blood tests was checking hormone levels to see if you are menopausal. He also thought that while blood was being taken, you should have some 'general MOT tests'.
- If asked, your mood swings and tiredness started 6 months ago. Little things, like someone leaving the toothpaste uncapped, upset you to the point of tears. You know that your reaction to minor issues is disproportional but you cannot seem to control your anger, irritation and hurt.
- You thought you were not coping with the added responsibility of studying nursing as a mature student so you discontinued the studies and took up a nursing assistant post at the hospice instead.
- You think your symptoms are due to 'stress'. Several issues cause 'stress': feeling lonely at home now that your second teenage daughter has left home to start university; doing menial, boring, repetitive housework; and dealing with dying people at work.
- Your husband, who is nine years younger than you, is busy working towards a promotion. You have spoken to him but feel that he has 'not listened'.
- If asked, you have not had regular periods; only occasional light bleeds since your endometrial ablation six months ago. This makes you feel even less of a woman. You also have hot flushes perhaps once or twice per week but you feel you can cope with them. However, you are tired, despite 8 hours of sleep, and would like to have more energy.
- If the doctor discusses HRT with you, you would like to know the pros and cons of HRT. You do not have contra-indications to HRT, but wonder if you are at increased risk of breast cancer as your mum's sister had breast cancer at age 52.
- If anti-depressants are discussed, you want to know if the doctor thinks 'it is all in my head'.
- You have come across alternative medications at the hospice and you are keen on 'natural remedies'. You would like more information on natural treatments for the menopause. You have read that phyto-oestrogens can be helpful but want the doctor's opinion.

Patient medical record for the doctor

Name   Kelly Carroll (46 years)

Past medical history   Endometrial ablation (6 months ago)
                                    Menorrhagia (2 years ago)
                                    Post-natal depression (9 years ago)

Past medication   zoladex implant 3.6 mg (6 months ago)

Consultation note by Dr Brown (4 weeks ago):
'Menopausal symptoms: hot flushes, feeling irritable, vaginal dryness, reduced energy and reduced sleep, waking early and ruminating. Has a stressful job at hospice. Finding it difficult not having periods after ablation. O/E: anxious lady with some pressure of speech. Near to tears at one point. Plan: for FSH, LH, progestogen and cholesterol bloods. ?menopause ?low mood worsening symptoms.'

Blood tests	Tests were done two weeks ago
Fasting glucose	6.2 (3–5.5)
Total cholesterol	6.5 mmol/l
HDL	1.2
Plasma oestradiol	42 pmol/l (40–1930)
Serum progestogen	1 mmol/l (14–90)
Plasma prolactin	77 mIU/l (60–620)
Plasma FSH	42 IU/l (1.5–33)
Plasma LH	32.5 IU/l (2–10)
TSH (2 years ago)	3.64 mIU/l (0.35–5.5)

Marking guide for the assessor

Generic indicators for targeted assessment domains	Descriptors – positive and negative
A. Data gathering, technical and assessment skills: • Gathering of data for clinical judgement, choice of examination, investigations and their interpretations. • Demonstrating proficiency in performing physical examinations and using diagnostic and therapeutic instruments.	Positive indicators: • Asks selective questions, tailored to establishing whether on balance, mood symptoms are most likely due to the menopause or to depression. • Enquires about red flags, such as deliberate self harm (DSH). Also takes an alcohol and drug history. • How the patient feels about the diagnosis and her commitment to different treatment options is explored in some depth. • Enquires about the raised isolated fasting blood glucose and explores possible causes. Negative indicators: • Questioning and mental state examination is not sufficiently selective. If red flags were present, the doctor would be more focused on safely treating depression. By excluding 'red flags', the doctor is able to offer a menu of treatment options. • The doctor fails to explore the patient's 'buy-in' to the diagnosis and consequently the issues arising from her preference for one treatment over an alternative is inadequately considered. • Details of the patient's family life and occupation are not obtained; the assessment is not holistic.

B. Clinical management skills	Positive indicators:
• Recognition and management of common medical conditions in primary care. Demonstrates flexible and structured approach to decision-making. • Demonstrating ability to deal with multiple complaints and co-morbidity and to promote a shared approach to managing problems.	• Doctors discuss what they feel are reasonable treatment options (ride it out, SSRIs, HRT, natural remedies) and explain their reasoning. • The pros and cons of the various management options are discussed. Information on HRT and breast cancer risk is explained in language the patient understands. • The patient is actively involved in the management plan and having obtained sufficient information from the doctor, makes an informed decision on treatment and follow-up. • Doctors arrange for appropriate investigation of the raised fasting glucose. Negative indicators: • Doctors fail to discuss treatment options in a manner that enables the patient to make informed decisions. Doctors may use jargon or technical language. • The patient is not managed safely or in line with current best practice. Some of the treatment options offered are unorthodox or unconventional to UK practice. • Follow-up arrangements are inadequate.

C. Interpersonal skills	Positive indicators:
<ul><li>Use of recognised communication techniques that enhance understanding of a patient's illness and promote a shared approach to managing problems.</li><li>Practising ethically with respect for equality and diversity in line with accepted codes of professional conduct.</li></ul>	<ul><li>The doctor displays empathy and understanding of how the patient's symptoms affect her relationships, work and self-perception.</li><li>The doctor communicates effectively – he or she addresses the specific concerns about HRT and breast cancer and the patient's reluctance to be viewed as a 'head case'.</li><li>The doctor fulfils the patient's expectation for advice about 'natural' menopausal remedies.</li><li>The doctor and patient develop a shared management plan – the patient buys in to the diagnosis and management.</li></ul> Negative indicators: <ul><li>The doctor fails to explore the patient's reluctance to accept a diagnosis of 'menopause'.</li><li>By failing to appreciate her desire to see this as a 'stress problem' to be treated by changing to a phyto-oestrogen rich diet, the doctor may be accused of 'medicalising' the issue and treating with 'pills'. The doctor behaves in a paternalistic manner.</li><li>The doctor appears judgemental or dismissive about the use of natural remedies, which seems at odds with the medical philosophy of the hospice at which she works.</li></ul>

Group debrief

Was the doctor able to complete his or her essential tasks? Did he or she safely and adequately manage the mood symptoms with sufficient patient involvement and did the doctor act on the isolated raised fasting glucose?

Discuss how the doctor could, if needed, improve his or her performance. In particular, assess whether the doctor:

- established rapport? If so, how?
- addressed Mrs Carroll's specific concerns about breast cancer and being perceived as a 'head case'? If so, how?
- addressed Mrs Carroll's expectations for information on natural remedies for the menopause?
- discussed the evidence base for HRT and natural remedies using simple and jargon-free language?
- involved the patient in the management plan?

Doctors with good interpersonal skills actively elicit the patient's ideas ('I am stressed. I don't think I'm menopausal – that means I'm old'; her concerns (If HRT will help me, how safe is it?') and expectations ('Could natural remedies be equally helpful?'). They incorporate the patient's beliefs into their management plan. If this patient did not buy in to the diagnosis of menopause, how likely is she to comply with a prescription for HRT or SSRIs? What is the harm associated in trying natural remedies for a short period of time? If the patient was not actively involved in the management plan, suggest how the consultation could be made more patient centred.

Relevant literature

http://www.emedicine.com/med/topic3756.htm

Practice case 15 – Pelvic pain and bleeding

Brief to the patient

- You are Kay Northrop, a 35 year old married bookkeeper. You attend today because you have had right and middle lower abdominal pain for three days. Although the pain is intermittent, the spasms develop and reach a peak (8/10) before subsiding to a dull ache. This pattern has occurred every few hours for the last three days and seems to be getting worse, rather than better. It does not feel like your IBS pain. You do not feel pregnant.
- The only other symptom is vaginal bleeding, which started 20 days ago. Initially you assumed this was your period, but the bleeding, though light, has continued, mainly in the form of spotting, requiring the use of a panty-liner. Your usual cycle is 4 to 6 days of bleeding every 30 days. You assumed you were bleeding for longer than usual because you missed two periods.
- You do not have urinary frequency, dysuria, diarrhoea or vomiting. You were able to eat today; no nausea or upset tummy.
- You think 'something is wrong' and suspect appendicitis or a miscarriage. You are worried about having a miscarriage. Your husband is in a meeting in Belfast. You are worried about calling him and disrupting his meeting if you have a minor ailment. On the other hand, you are scared about having a miscarriage or being admitted into hospital without him.
- You expect to be told what is wrong with you, how serious it is and how it should be treated. You need sufficient information to decide whether you should ask your husband to shorten his business trip and return home tonight.
- When you saw Dr Brown 3 weeks ago, you were advised to have a blood test 7 days before your next period was due but you started bleeding two days later, so the test was not done.
- If the doctor asks to test your urine, you produce a piece of paper: 'Urine pregnancy test positive. Dipstix: trace leucocytes but no nitrites or protein'.
- If the doctor offers to perform a pelvic examination, you decline (you don't want to be examined while bleeding) unless absolutely necessary. If the doctor convinces you that by examining you, he or she will be able to make a diagnosis, you permit the examination and produce a card: 'Os closed. Tender in right adnexa but no mass palpated. No peritonism'.
- If the doctor checks your pulse and BP, you produce a card: 'pulse 84 regular; BP 132/88'.

Patient medical record for the doctor

Name   Kay Northrop (35 years)

Social and family history Married 2 years ago. No children

Past medical history   Pre-pregnancy counselling (3 weeks ago)
           Irritable bowel syndrome (3 months ago)

Past medication   Mebeverine 135mg thrice daily × 100T (3 months ago)

Consultation note by Dr Brown (3 weeks ago):
'Stopped Microgynon 12 months ago. Actively trying for a baby for past 8 months. LMP: three months ago. Missed last two periods and then has a bleed lasting 24 hours. After the second missed period, two pregnancy tests were negative. Recent blood tests, including hormone profile, were fine. No past history of STIs or pelvic infection or surgery. Plan: get 21 day progestogen. In view of age (and husband is 38; neither have had children) refer to fertility clinic at next appointment.'

Answers to Case 9

1. False – the pain is usually caused by collagen or muscle origin fascia at the medial tubercle of the calcaneus
2. True
3. False – patients often notice pain at the begin...eroid injections relieve symptoms fairly quickly, they warm up
4. False – patients with pes planus (low arches ...owed no benefit over placebo at increased risk for developing plantar fascii...in tennis elbow and related conditions
5. True
6. True
7. False – with age, running shoes lose a signific... getting a new pair of shoes may be helpful in ...rs, after which active movement is encouraged
8. True

Answers to Case 10

1. True – anabolic steroids improve nitrogen ut... balance by the reversal of the catabolic proce... are sprained ankles a state of chronic catabolism
2. False – oral anabolic-androgenic steroids are... cessation, and their metabolites can be clear... has been detected in the urine of an athlete 4... nandrolone (an injectable anabolic-androge...pecificity is around 25% up to 2 years after last reported use ...ose
3. True
4. True – insulin resistance and diminished glu... powerlifters
5. True – anabolic-androgenic steroids have tra...id purine-rich foods, such as liver, kidneys and often using more than one steroid at a time (...are not a problem, see: http://arthritis.about. moving from low starting doses to higher do... the end of the cycle ...on with allopurinol if a person is having two or
6. True – they appear to increase arousal, self-...

Answers to Case 11

1. True   ...an acute attack of gout
2. False – the WHO classifies anaemia in pregn...
3. False – if iron deficiency anaemia co-exists w... distribution width (RDW) is increased
4. True
5. True   ...ent
6. False – a 125 g can of sardines in tomato sau... lean roast beef   ...eovessel formation, collagen fibre disarray, but
7. False – a 30 g bowl of branflakes contains thr... cornflakes   ...el-drop exercises, GTN patches, sclerosing
                                           ...While peritendinous corticosteroid injections
                                           ...s, they have no long-term effects.

Marking guide for the assessor

Generic indicators for targeted assessment domains	Descriptors – positive and negative
A. Data gathering, technical and assessment skills: • Gathering of data for clinical judgement, choice of examination, investigations and their interpretations. • Demonstrating proficiency in performing physical examinations and using diagnostic and therapeutic instruments.	Positive indicators: • Asks open questions (to explore the nature of the pelvic pain and bleeding) followed by closed questions to clarify LMP and sequence of events. • Asks about red flags: obtains information to assess if this could be a miscarriage, ectopic pregnancy or appendicitis. • If hypovolaemic shock were found on examination, it would add weight to an emergency presentation of ectopic pregnancy. The normal pulse and BP are reassuring. • The most important examination is the pregnancy test. There are arguments for and against performing a vaginal examination (VE). Consider whether performing a VE in a suspected miscarriage or ectopic pregnancy contributes much to the clinical picture. Negative indicators: • Does not systematically gather data from history or examination; makes assumptions about the problem. • Not appropriately selective in choice of examination. • Fails to interpret examination findings correctly.

Group debrief

The most common reason for failure in the CSA is the candidate's failure to dev
management plan. This case tests the candidate's ability to recognise and mana
case of pelvic pain and vaginal bleeding. The differential diagnosis includes ble
in an early normal pregnancy; however, it is difficult to exclude a miscarriage o
ectopic pregnancy on clinical grounds. Also, the patient's social support is mini
The doctor needs to suspect an ectopic pregnancy (red flag), broach the possib
bad news, support her and deal with the emergency.

Discuss how the doctor could, if needed, improve his or her performance. In
particular, assess whether the doctor:

- identified the patient's problem with an appropriate opening question, e.g. '
  can I do for you today?'
- established dates and sequence of events
- encouraged the patient to express her feelings?
- demonstrated appropriate confidence?
- assessed the patient's prior knowledge before giving information and gave
  explanations after discovering the extent of patient's wish for information?
- checked with the patient whether plans were accepted and if concerns were
  addressed?
- explained seriousness, expected outcome, short- and long-term consequenc
- safety-netted by explaining possible unexpected outcomes and clarified whe
  how to seek help?

This case specifically tests the doctor's ability to develop a safe, evidence-based
management plan. Bearing this in mind, assess whether the doctor was able to
establish a differential diagnosis, recognise the need for further investigation an
arrange for appropriate help within the allocated time?

Relevant literature

For an overview of the management of bleeding in early pregnancy, see:
Rawal N *et al.* (2009) Bleeding in early pregnancy. *InnovAiT*, **2 (5):** 277–283.
doi:10.1093/innovait/inp053

RCOG (2004, revised 2010) The management of tubal pregnancy. Green Top
Guideline – www.rcog.org.uk/files/rcog-corp/GTG21_230611.pdf.

Answers to Case 12

1. True
2. False – about 90% of the risk for bowel cancer is thought to be due to dietary factors
3. False – trials have shown that the risk can be reduced by almost 50%
4. True – HNPCC is inherited as an autosomal dominant; familial polyposis coli accounts for 1% of cases
5. False – a single FOB is negative with up to 50% of cancers; the figure is about 30% if done on 3 consecutive days
6. True – refer to the July 2000 two week referral guidelines

Answers to Case 13

1. False – diarrhoea, cramping, abdominal pain, and fever within 2–5 days after exposure to the organism are symptoms of campylobacteriosis
2. False – some patients with campylobacteriosis may be asymptomatic
3. False – campylobacteriosis is often associated with the consumption of undercooked meat (especially poultry), unpasteurized milk, or untreated water
4. True
5. True
6. True
7. False – loperamide should be avoided in people with severe symptoms or dysentery because of the risk of precipitating ileus or toxic megacolon

Answers to Case 14

1. False – approximately 80% are asymptomatic
2. True
3. False – bacterial orchitis rarely occurs without an associated epididymitis and unilateral testicular oedema occurs in 90% of cases
4. True
5. True

Answers to Case 15

1. False – enuresis is the involuntary discharge of urine by day or night or both, in a child aged 5 years or older, in the absence of congenital or acquired defects of the nervous system or urinary tract
2. False – as many as 70% of children with nocturnal enuresis have a positive family history of childhood bedwetting
3. True
4. True
5. True
6. True
7. False – the only investigations required in primary nocturnal enuresis are urinalysis and urine culture to exclude diabetes mellitus and a urinary tract infection

8. False – do not restrict fluids; the child should have about eight drinks a day, spaced out throughout the day, the last one about 1 hour before bed
9. False – enuresis alarms, the first-line treatment in motivated children over 7 years, come in vibrating or sound modes; the vibrating alarm is preferable in children who share rooms or who are deaf
10. True

Answers to Case 16

1. True
2. True
3. False – it doubles the relative risk
4. True
5. False – NICE guidelines: localised intermediate risk prostate cancer can be treated with radical surgery, radical radiotherapy or active surveillance. Men with high risk localised cancer should be offered radical prostatectomy or external beam radiotherapy. Hormonal treatment is not routinely recommended for men with biochemical relapse after radical treatment unless they also have symptomatic local disease progression, or proven metastases, or a PSA level that has doubled in less than 3 months.

Answers to Case 17

1. False – dyspnoea, chest pain, or haemoptysis are symptoms of pulmonary embolism
2. False – a positive Homan's sign is pain in the calf or popliteal region on passive abrupt, forceful dorsiflexion of the ankle with the knee in a flexed position.
3. True
4. True
5. False – D-dimer assays are more sensitive for proximal than distal DVT, probably because proximal thromboses have a greater volume than distal thromboses
6. False – D-dimer levels can fall significantly after heparin is given
7. False – repeat ultrasonography is indicated in people with a negative initial ultrasound if they are at moderate to high risk for DVT and the D-dimer test was positive
8. False – one of the differential diagnoses of a DVT is a ruptured Baker's cyst, which is a cyst that forms in the popliteal fossa from an outpouching of synovial membrane of the knee joint

Answers to Case 18

1. False – 81% are venous
2. True
3. False – skin pigmentation and varicose veins suggest a venous cause, while cold, shiny hairless skin suggests an arterial cause
4. True
5. False – ulcers should be cleaned by gentle irrigation to prevent damaging the wound bed

6. False – graduated compression bandages should not be used if the ABPI suggests significant arterial disease
7. True – these patients may require surgery or angiography
8. False – antibiotics have little effect on wound healing and should not be used to treat organisms that have colonised a wound that are not causing clinical signs or symptoms of infection

Answers to Case 19

1. True
2. False – hoarseness due to hypothyroidism is unlikely to resolve with thyroxine treatment
3. True
4. False – if hoarseness persists for more than 6 weeks, refer to an ENT surgeon to inspect the vocal cords to exclude oropharyngeal malignancy
5. False – the effect of inhaled steroids on hoarseness is dose-related

Answers to Case 20

1. False – a 2-week washout period is required
2. True
3. True
4. True
5. False – UK prevalence is just under 30%

Marking guide for the assessor

Generic indicators for targeted assessment domains	Descriptors – positive and negative
A. Data gathering, technical and assessment skills: • Gathering of data for clinical judgement, choice of examination, investigations and their interpretations. • Demonstrating proficiency in performing physical examinations and using diagnostic and therapeutic instruments.	Positive indicators: • Asks open questions (to explore the nature of the pelvic pain and bleeding) followed by closed questions to clarify LMP and sequence of events. • Asks about red flags: obtains information to assess if this could be a miscarriage, ectopic pregnancy or appendicitis. • If hypovolaemic shock were found on examination, it would add weight to an emergency presentation of ectopic pregnancy. The normal pulse and BP are reassuring. • The most important examination is the pregnancy test. There are arguments for and against performing a vaginal examination (VE). Consider whether performing a VE in a suspected miscarriage or ectopic pregnancy contributes much to the clinical picture. Negative indicators: • Does not systematically gather data from history or examination; makes assumptions about the problem. • Not appropriately selective in choice of examination. • Fails to interpret examination findings correctly.

B. Clinical management skills	Positive indicators:
• Recognition and management of common medical conditions in primary care. Demonstrates flexible and structured approach to decision-making. • Demonstrating ability to deal with multiple complaints and co-morbidity and to promote a shared approach to managing problems.	• The doctor explains the most likely causes of vaginal bleeding with pain in early pregnancy (bleeding in early normal pregnancy / miscarriage / ectopic) in jargon-free language. • Management options, including same or next day appointment in Early Pregnancy Unit (EPU), with early blood tests or scanning, are openly discussed. • Management, including what to do if the pain or bleeding worsens, is discussed. The patient is given sufficient information about best and worst case scenarios to decide on whether or not she interrupts her husband's business trip. Negative indicators: • Doctors fail to consider common conditions in the differential diagnosis or fail to explain these conditions sufficiently to enhance the patient's understanding. • Further investigation and management is not selective. • Decisions about referral are inappropriate or ill timed. • Safety-netting or follow-up arrangements are inadequate.

C. Interpersonal skills	Positive indicators:
• Use of recognised communication techniques that enhance understanding of a patient's illness and promote a shared approach to managing problems. • Practising ethically with respect for equality and diversity in line with accepted codes of professional conduct.	• The doctor explores the patient's agenda; he or she identifies the patient's ideas about miscarriage or appendicitis; her concerns about being alone in hospital and her expectations for sufficient information to recall her husband if needed. • The doctor explores the patient's ambivalence to VE; is empathetic, non-judgemental and respectful when discussing this with her. He or she provides an explanation of why the examination is chosen/not chosen. • The doctor discusses what he or she feels is the safest action (same or next day appointment in the EPU). However, if the patient expresses a strong preference for being assessed at a later date, when her husband is present, he or she negotiates with the patient to construct a shared management plan, which includes good safety-netting. Negative indicators: • Doctors fail to share their thoughts about the possible diagnosis and the need to manage risk well. The patient is not provided with sufficient information to be meaningfully involved in making decisions. • The doctor seems frustrated or irritated by the patient's reluctance to have a VE and responds negatively. • The doctor instructs the patient; the patient's wishes are not explored or considered in the management decisions.

Group debrief

The most common reason for failure in the CSA is the candidate's failure to develop a management plan. This case tests the candidate's ability to recognise and manage a case of pelvic pain and vaginal bleeding. The differential diagnosis includes bleeding in an early normal pregnancy; however, it is difficult to exclude a miscarriage or an ectopic pregnancy on clinical grounds. Also, the patient's social support is minimal. The doctor needs to suspect an ectopic pregnancy (red flag), broach the possibility of bad news, support her and deal with the emergency.

Discuss how the doctor could, if needed, improve his or her performance. In particular, assess whether the doctor:
- identified the patient's problem with an appropriate opening question, e.g. 'What can I do for you today?'
- established dates and sequence of events
- encouraged the patient to express her feelings?
- demonstrated appropriate confidence?
- assessed the patient's prior knowledge before giving information and gave explanations after discovering the extent of patient's wish for information?
- checked with the patient whether plans were accepted and if concerns were addressed?
- explained seriousness, expected outcome, short- and long-term consequences?
- safety-netted by explaining possible unexpected outcomes and clarified when and how to seek help?

This case specifically tests the doctor's ability to develop a safe, evidence-based management plan. Bearing this in mind, assess whether the doctor was able to establish a differential diagnosis, recognise the need for further investigation and arrange for appropriate help within the allocated time?

Relevant literature

For an overview of the management of bleeding in early pregnancy, see:
Rawal N *et al.* (2009) Bleeding in early pregnancy. *InnovAiT*, **2 (5):** 277–283. doi:10.1093/innovait/inp053

RCOG (2004, revised 2010) The management of tubal pregnancy. Green Top Guideline – www.rcog.org.uk/files/rcog-corp/GTG21_230611.pdf.

Answers to "Test your theoretical knowledge" questions

Answers to Case 1

1. False – for vasomotor symptoms, consider a 2 week trial of paroxetine (20 mg daily)
2. True
3. False – Venlafaxine 37.5 mg twice a day is unlicensed for the treatment of menopausal flushing
4. True
5. False – ginseng, black cohosh, and red clover have oestrogenic properties and should not be used in women with contraindications to oestrogen (e.g. breast cancer)

Answers to Case 2

1. True
2. False – NICE guidelines require all of a list of criteria to be fulfilled before bariatric surgery can be recommended
3. True
4. False – NICE does not recommend use of bioimpedance, however, the National Obesity Forum guidelines do
5. True
6. True

Answers to Case 3

1. True
2. True
3. False – leave-on emollients should be prescribed in large quantities (250–500 g weekly)
4. True
5. False – NICE recommends that healthcare professionals review repeat prescriptions of products for children with atopic eczema at least once a year
6. False – topical tacrolimus is recommended, within its licensed indications, as an option for the second-line treatment of moderate to severe atopic eczema, in adults and children aged 2 years and older, that has not been controlled by topical corticosteroids
7. True
8. False – healthcare professionals should offer a 7–14 day trial of an age-appropriate sedating antihistamine to children aged 6 months or over during an acute flare of atopic eczema if sleep disturbance has a significant impact on the child or parents or carers

Answers to Case 4

1. False – it involves the common extensor muscle origin
2. True
3. True
4. False – trials have shown that corticosteroid injections relieve symptoms fairly quickly, but that this is not long-lasting
5. False – a multicentre European trial showed no benefit over placebo
6. True – some trials have shown benefit in tennis elbow and related conditions
7. True – both increase the torque and vibration the arm receives

Answers to Case 5

1. False – rest sprained ankles for 48 hours, after which active movement is encouraged
2. True
3. False – advise patients to improve balance by practising balancing on the injured leg with the eyes shut, once the pain has settled
4. True
5. False – more than 75% of ankle injuries are sprained ankles

Answers to Case 6

1. True
2. True
3. False – sensitivity is around 90%, but specificity is around 25%
4. True – but CT has a higher radiation dose
5. True – see 2007 Cochrane Review

Answers to Case 7

1. False – advise patients with gout to avoid purine-rich foods, such as liver, kidneys and seafood; bananas, chocolate and tuna are not a problem, see: http://arthritis.about.com/od/gout/a/foodstoeat.htm
2. False – consider prophylactic medication with allopurinol if a person is having two or more attacks of gout in a year
3. True
4. True
5. False – do not stop allopurinol during an acute attack of gout

Answers to Case 8

1. True – quinolones
2. True
3. False – both these features may be absent
4. True
5. False – there is hypervascularity with neovessel formation, collagen fibre disarray, but inflammatory cells are absent
6. False – evidence supports the use of heel-drop exercises, GTN patches, sclerosing injections and microcurrent therapy. While peritendinous corticosteroid injections have short-term pain-relieving benefits, they have no long-term effects.